HOW TO SAVE YOUR LOVED ONES FROM COVID

Early Treatment is the Key

Michael Arnold, MD, L.Ac.

MYSTERY DANCE PRESS
Aptos, California USA

First Edition May 2021
Print ISBN 978-1-7321041-1-2
E-book ISBN 978-1-7321041-2-9
Front cover photo: Marcin Jozwiak

Published by
Mystery Dance Press
PO Box 1359
Capitola, CA, USA
http://michaelarnoldmdlac.com

DISCLAIMER

This document is prepared for informational purposes only. It is not intended as a substitute for competent medical care from a healthcare professional. It is not intended to be a way to delay getting needed medical treatment.

But whether or not you have access to proper medical care, the more you know the better things will go if you or a loved one gets in a challenging situation.

Every effort has been made toward having this information be complete, up-to-date, and accurate. However, I cannot guarantee such. This is especially so since our knowledge around Covid is so rapidly changing.

Finally, please understand that much of this document contains my medical opinion. That opinion is based on my training, my three post-graduate degrees, my research and my over forty years of experience treating patients in clinic. These opinions are shared by many other highly qualified physicians. There is a spectrum of opinion on this hotly-debated subject. You have both the freedom and the responsibility of deciding where you stand in that debate.

TABLE OF CONTENTS

APPENDICES

Introduction

Early treatment is the key to being safe from COVID-19. Ivermectin is the most effective early treatment at this time. The medical system has, in some ways, failed us. COVID-19 is a new, fast-moving, fast-changing illness. Modern medicine is a slow-moving, gargantuan orthodoxy, encrusted with complex rules and procedures and severely corrupted by the profit motives of Big Pharma.

The purpose of this manual is to prepare you with specific recommendations regarding:

- What resources to have ready and on-hand in case someone falls ill with COVID-19. Get these in advance!
- What to do in case of COVID-19.

None of these recommendations (at the time of this writing - April, 2021) are endorsed by the CDC, the FDA nor any of the major medical societies in the United States (such as the American Academy of Family Practice or the American Board of Internal Medicine).

In fact, here is what the CDC has to say if you actually have COVID-19:

"**Take care of yourself.** Get rest and stay hydrated. Take over-the-counter medicines, such as acetaminophen, to help you feel better." (https://www.cdc.gov/coronavirus/2019-ncov/if-you-are-sick/steps-when-sick.html). That's it. End of advice.

In the world of the CDC, there is nothing else you can do until you become so sick that you have to go to the Emergency Room, go on oxygen, and possibly go on a ventilator.

Yet many, many highly-qualified physicians feel strongly that an inexpensive drug called Ivermectin (as well as many other things) can indeed help prevent and treat COVID-19 (**APPENDIX 3: Knowledgable Experts**).

The time to build the levees is before the flood. Prepare now. If you or a loved one do fall seriously ill, you will have neither the time nor the energy necessary to help yourself with the protocols in this manual. For this reason, I have included **APPENDIX 8: Shopping List for COVID-19 Preparedness**.

Why Has Ivermectin Been Suppressed?

Ivermectin is an antibiotic which can help with COVID-19. Hundreds of medical papers attest to this. Many of us healthcare providers are heartbroken by what we see as the systematic censoring and suppression of all treatments or cures for COVID-19 outside of a narrow, highly profitable window of vaccines and costly new drugs. From our point of view, people are suffering and dying unnecessarily because of this.

While I have followed the COVID-19 epidemic closely since the beginning, the matter came to a head for me when a certain video was taken down off YouTube. This video showed a United States Senate fact-finding panel questioning a licensed, Board-Certified Medical Doctor about the use of a common, inexpensive medicine called Ivermectin to treat COVID-19.

The physician was very sincere. He said they were getting wonderful results. Then he said what, to me, were the magic words – "I'm not asking you to adopt the treatment. I'm simply asking you to go review the evidence on the subject."

Now in my world, when a media giant takes down a video of a United States Senator and a board-certified physician having a reasonable conversation about a therapy, we have a big, big problem. In the time of shut-down, when "in public" means on digital media platforms, our right to free speech has been taken away. If we don't leap to the defense of that freedom, then we don't deserve to have it. Going, going, gone.

The physician was Pierre Kory, MD, former Chief of the Critical Care Service and Medical Director of the Trauma and Life Support Center at the University of Wisconsin, Board Certified in Internal Medicine and Certified in both Pulmonary Diseases and Critical Care Medicine. In the hierarchy of medical doctors, this gentleman is way up there.

In developing the FLCCC protocols, Dr. Kory worked with a number of other highly trained and qualified physicians, including Paul Marik, MD, Professor of Medicine and Chief of Pulmonary and Critical Care Medicine at the Eastern Virginia Medical School. He heads a department at a medical school, and he has extensive credentials.

So I downloaded his position paper, titled "EVMS COVID-19 Management" from:

https://www.evms.edu/media/evmspublic/departments/internalmedicine/EVMSCriticalCareCOVID-19Protocol.pdf.

Updates to the protocol can be found on the website of the FLCCC (Front Line COVID-19 Critical Care Alliance):

https://COVID19criticalcare.com/math-hospital-treatment/.

In addition, if you would like to review the 464 references in their bibliography you can find it at

https://COVID19criticalcare.com/wp-content/uploads/2020/12/FLCCC-Protocols-—-A-Guide-to-the-Management-of-COVID-19.pdf

Once I had the document, I dove into the laborious process of reviewing many of the more than 460 scientific papers listed in the bibliography. And while there is no certainty in science or medicine, **I am convinced that the weight of the evidence supports my medical opinion: the potential benefits of the Ivermectin approach far outweigh the risks.** Having arrived at that opinion, and in a time of censorship and suppression, I have an obligation to speak out.

Until recently, I was utterly mystified by the frantic and blatant efforts to suppress any development of a readily available, inexpensive treatment for COVID-19. Then, just a few days ago, some of the pieces fell into place. The California gold rush was, financially, a little blip when compared to the rush for a COVID-19 vaccine. Hundreds of billions, if not trillions, of dollars are at stake. But under **the U.S. law of Emergency Use Authorization**, all of these profits will vanish in an instant if one single treatment for COVID-19 by an already-existing medicine is approved.

It's a point of law. The "Emergency Use Authorization of Medical Products and Related Authorities" guidance statement issued by the federal government (https://www.fda.gov/media/97321/download) puts it as follows:

(Under section B, Item 1. "Criteria for Issuance of EUA," sub-section d):

"No Alternatives For FDA to issue an EUA

"**There must be no adequate, approved, and available alternative to the candidate product** for diagnosing, preventing, or treating the disease or condition."

So if one single "adequate, approved, and available" treatment for COVID-19 is found, all the vaccine manufacturers instantly lose their Emergency Use Authorization. They can no longer rush a dangerous, untested, experimental vaccine to market. They would have to take these new vaccines through the standard evaluation and safety testing normally required by the FDA. This usually takes seven or eight years. The vaccine manufacturers would lose billions and billions in potential income.

As they say in the murder mysteries,
"Follow the money."

If you think all this might even possibly be true, don't you have a responsibility to investigate and find out for yourself? If you find out it is true, don't you have a responsibility to stand up and speak out?

The Ivermectin Protocol

This manual advocates a simple form of the Ivermectin-based approach developed by the Front Line Critical Care COVID-19 Alliance ("FLCCC"):

https://COVID19criticalcare.com/

Ivermectin is an inexpensive drug which has already been found safe and has been fully approved by the FDA for other purposes.

Another antibiotic that has been re-purposed for COVID-19 is Hydroxychloroquine. However, Hydroxychloroquine is for the most part only useful for early COVID-19 in high-risk patients. Ivermectin has broader applicability, so Ivermectin is my focus. The Hydroxycholoquine-based approach is described briefly in **APPENDIX 9: The HCQ (Hydroxychloroquine) Approach**.

If you decide you want Ivermectin on-hand, it may take a little time and effort to obtain it. Get some Ivermectin now. It's better to have it and not need it than to need it and not have it. For avenues to Ivermectin, please see **APPENDIX 2: Obtaining Ivermectin**.

Part One
Overview

CHAPTER 1

Working With the Stages of COVID-19

I see four basic stages of dealing with COVID-19. Different actions are needed at each stage.

1. Staying Healthy. In this book I describe the medicines and supplements that we can take to prevent serious COVID-19.

Of course, the real work of staying healthy is much more far-reaching. Staying healthy requires intentional cultivation in many areas of life, including:

- Learning how to stay healthy
- Cultivating a positive state of mind
- Connecting with others in a healthy way
- Deep breathing
- Movement/exercise
- Diet
- Good sleep
- Being in nature

... *and much much more*

If you would like to go further into my point of view on staying healthy and strong, have a look at my website:

http://www.michaelarnoldmdlac.com/

Also, I give a weekly Zoom called "***In the Palace of Health,***" where the focus is entirely on getting and staying healthy. It's a fun and positive space (You can sign up through my website).

2. Got exposed: What to do if you know you have been exposed to someone who has COVID-19. You think they may have given it to you (They call this "*Post-Exposure Prophylaxis*").

3. COVID-19 with Symptoms: How to recognize if you have actually come down with COVID-19, and how to respond to that situation (They call this "*Early Outpatient COVID-19.*")

4. Severe COVID-19: How to recognize if COVID-19 has become serious and is beginning to incite the severe, destructive reaction called the cytokine storm. When to go to the ER or call 911.

CHAPTER 2

Should I Get Tested for COVID-19?

My opinion is: Don't bother. I consider the PCR test unsound and unreliable. I arrived at this conclusion after looking deeply into the science behind it. Even the inventor of the PCR test, Kary Mullis, Ph.D., was adamant that the PCR test cannot be used to diagnose disease. (https://www.youtube.com/watch?v=rXm9kAhNj-4) That is not the purpose for which it is designed. Dr. Mullis, by the way, was awarded a Nobel Prize for his work in discovering the PCR test.

That the tests, especially the PCR tests, are unreliable is one of the main reasons that there are no real, reliable statistics around this epidemic.

From my point of view tests for COVID-19 usually only serve to create a delay while you wait for the results. Delay in treatment is not acceptable. All the experts who feel that COVID-19 can actually be treated agree on one thing: **early treatment is the key**.

Part Two
The Ivermectin-Based Protocol

CHAPTER 3

Staying Healthy

The Four Supplements that Make it Highly Unlikely You Will Fall Seriously Ill

There are four core supplements that make it very unlikely that you could fall seriously ill should you contract COVID-19. They are:

- **Zinc —50 mg/day**
- **Vitamin D—1,000 to 3,000/day**
- **Vitamin C—1,000 mg twice daily**
- **Quercetin—250 mg/day**

If you do nothing more than take these four inexpensive, readily available supplements every day, you drastically reduce your chances of falling ill from COVID-19.

The Rationale for These Specific Supplements

We see a bewildering array of supplements and advice about supplements. I have focused on these four to keep it simple.

ZINC: The virus which causes COVID-19 is an RNA

virus. When the RNA gets into our cells, it hijacks the cell's machinery to build more virus particles. The virus does this by first tricking our cells into making an enzyme that makes more COVID-19 RNA. **Zinc blocks this enzyme.** (This enzyme is called "*RNA-dependent RNA polymerase*".)

Also, Zinc is essential to the proper functioning of the immune system in general. It has been taken for the common cold for quite some time.

Zinc deficiency is very common, and figuring out whether or not someone is actually deficient in Zinc is not so simple. So please be safe; take Zinc.

VITAMIN D: There is a strong association between low Vitamin D and severe COVID-19.

In one study Vitamin D deficiency was found in 82% of COVID-19 cases and 47% of the population at large. (https://academic.oup.com/jcem/advance-article/doi/10.1210/clinem/dgaa733/5934827) This tells us that your risk of getting a bad case of COVID-19 skyrockets when you are vitamin D deficient.It also shows that Vitamin D deficiency is very, very common (almost half of the population in this study).

Vitamin D is essential to the healthy function of the immune system. There is extensive research that shows if you have good levels of Vitamin D, you are less likely to get any viral infection of the lungs or upper airways. There is even evidence showing that people are less likely to get tuberculosis if they have healthy levels of Vitamin D.

But taking a bunch of Vitamin D all of a sudden when you are already ill doesn't work very well. It's important to take Vitamin D regularly to get the protective effect.

It's possible to overdose on Vitamin D, so if you want to go above the doses recommended here, I would do some more research or talk to a knowledgeable expert first. I know several nutritionists who say that higher doses are perfectly safe.

"You cannot get the cytokine storm if you have a normal Vitamin D level." – Ryan Cole, MD (https://www.bitchute.com/video/nAWbvsCBM2JG/)

VITAMIN C: So much has been published about Vitamin C and its beneficial effects that I feel no further comment is needed. It is scary to note that YouTube and Facebook have taken down information on the beneficial effects of Vitamin C for COVID-19.

"I have not seen any flu yet that was not cured or markedly ameliorated by massive doses of vitamin C."
– Robert F. Cathcart, MD

QUERCETIN: Quercetin is a natural pigment present in many fruits, vegetables and grains. Quercetin is generally beneficial for the immune system and inflammation. In addition, there is one specific thing Quercetin does which is very important in short-circuiting COVID-19's attack. Quercetin helps Zinc get inside our cells.

As you read above, Zinc is key in stopping COVID-19 because it jams up the machinery by which COVID-19 reproduces inside our cells. But even if you take Zinc, it doesn't necessarily get into the cell. The cell membrane stops the Zinc from getting in. Quercetin helps the Zinc get into the cell so that the Zinc can be effective.

(This, by the way, is one of the ways that Hydroxychloroquine also helps against COVID-19.)

Quercetin has many other beneficial functions. Like Zinc, Quercetin enters our cells and interferes with the functioning of the COVID-19 virus. Also, two of the most serious manifestations of the cytokine storm are inflammation and clotting. Quercetin reduces inflammation and inhibits clotting.

MELATONIN: The FLCCC also recommends Melatonin 6 mg near bedtime, but I have reservations:

In this context Melatonin is being used to keep down inflammation in the body, since the more inflammation a person is carrying around before they get COVID-19, the more likely they are to suffer the cytokine storm. After all, inflammation is simply intense activation of the immune system. And believe me, a lot of people are carrying around a lot of inflammation in this world. Inflammation from state of mind, from diet, from toxic environments, and more.

Yet I am not enthusiastic about using Melatonin regularly, and here is why: Melatonin is a messenger molecule that your brain secretes when it's dark. It tells the body it's time to wind down and sleep. Until recently, Melatonin was known mainly as a sleep aid. As it turns out, Melatonin has many healing and anti-inflammatory actions in the body. It makes sense. When do we do a great deal of our healing and reducing of inflammation? While we are at rest in the night.

But here's the thing: Your body should naturally secrete Melatonin. If you always give it Melatonin, little by little the body's ability to secrete Melatonin on its own will dwindle. It's like muscles - if you don't work them, they atrophy.

I recommend instead good sleep hygiene and providing the circumstances by which a healthy amount of Melatonin would be secreted by the brain every night. That would involve things like keeping the electronics out of your bedroom, having your room dark at night, no staring at screens within a couple of hours of bedtime, and so on.

Of course, if you actually have an active COVID-19 infection, go ahead and take Melatonin 10 mg near bedtime every night for a couple of weeks or so. Then, when things are getting back to normal, let your brain cells resume doing their job. They need the work.

CHAPTER 4

High Risk Individuals

"Prophylaxis for High Risk Individuals"

Take the supplement regimen described in Chapter 3 above–**Staying Healthy**.

Add **IVERMECTIN**:

- For the average adult the dose is 12 mg.
- If your weight is not near average, then the dose is 0.1 mg/lb (which is the same as 0.2 mg/kg).

  one dose to start

  2nd dose in 48 hours,

  then one dose every 2 weeks

(For more details see **APPENDIX 1: Making Friends with Ivermectin**.)

Am I High Risk?

Should I take Ivermectin Just in Case?

Serious illness from COVID-19 most often occurs in people who are weak and in poor health. When a person has other medical conditions such as diabetes, high blood pressure, lung disease, heart disease, obesity and so on, the risk of becoming seriously ill from COVID-19 goes up.

The weaker and more seriously ill you are, the more you should consider taking a low dose of Ivermectin on a regular basis. This is called *prophylaxis*.

We don't really have a COVID-19 epidemic, even if you believe the statistics. We have an epidemic of chronic degenerative diseases of the metabolism, such as diabetes, heart disease, obesity and so on. We have an epidemic of toxins in our environment and our food. We have an epidemic of of people living with their bodies in a state of severe inflammation. Given the poor health of our nation, something was going to come along and start carrying the most afflicted away. If it wasn't COVID-19 it would have been something else.

For healthy people under the age of 60, I do not recommend taking Ivermectin "just in case." Please remember that if you are healthy and strong your risk of suffering from a COVID-19 infection is very, very low. Your body just shrugs off the illness. In fact, the virus that causes COVID-19 is from the Coronavirus family of viruses. Coronaviruses in general are one of the four most common causes of the common cold. We don't need to fear or flee from these everyday challenges to the immune system if we are healthy.

CHAPTER 5

Got Exposed to COVID-19

"Post COVID-19 Exposure Prophylaxis"

Continue the basic regimen of supplements from Section 1 (Zinc, Vitamin D, Vitamin C, Quercetin).

If you have not already been taking "Ivermectin for high risk individuals," take:

- **Ivermectin** 0.2 mg/kg per dose (Please see **APPENDIX 1: Making Friends with Ivermectin** to figure out what that comes to. For the average adult that is 12 mg.)
- 2nd dose in 48 hours
- That's it. Stop.

If you are already taking Ivermectin for high risk individuals, simply continue on as before.

If you are concerned that you have been exposed to COVID-19, resting and staying warm is fundamental. If you allow your immune system the space and resources, it will surely overcome this relatively low-risk virus. If you insist on pushing on through your life even though you feel tired and worn down, you are much more likely to fall ill.

CHAPTER 6

I Have COVID-19, But It's Not Too Bad

"Early Outpatient Protocol" or

"Symptomatic Patients at Home"

1. Take Ivermectin:

- Ivermectin 0.2 mg/kg of body weight per dose (which is the same as 0.1 mg/lb)
  (Please see **APPENDIX 1: Making Friends with Ivermectin** for help with that. The usual adult dose ends up being 12 mg.)
- One dose daily
- Minimum of 2 days
- Take until recovered, but no longer than five days.

2. Intensify and enhance the basic supplement regimen to:

- **Vitamin D3**: 4,000 IU/day
- **Vitamin C**: 2,000 mg 2–3 times daily (Caution – at higher doses, Vitamin C can cause digestive upset and loose stools.)
- **Quercetin**: 250 mg twice a day
- **Zinc**: 100 mg/day in divided doses (only for a few days. May cause stomach upset).

add

- **Aspirin:** 325 mg/day (unless contraindicated)
- **Melatonin:** 10 mg near bedtime until better.

3. Check Vitals 2 or 3 times daily—especially blood oxygen saturation with Pulse Oximeter (APPENDIX 4: Buying and Using the Pulse Oximeter).

4. Do things to prevent clotting:

See "Doing things to prevent clotting" (see p. 42)

How Would You Know If You Have COVID-19?

(i.e. When to start the "*Early Outpatient Protocol.*")

To navigate a COVID-19 scenario we need to rely, at least at first, on the information we can gather immediately while we are at home.

Prompt treatment is the key to success in treating COVID-19, so promptly figuring out when you may well have COVID-19 is very important. It is also very important to know immediately when COVID-19 has gone from mild to severe, because at that time the treatment changes and it's time to seek medical help.

Starting the "Early Outpatient Protocol" is not a big deal. You are not crossing the Rubicon or doing something irreversible like having your gallbladder removed. If you are at high risk for serious illness from COVID-19, it's better to start the regimen and turn out not to need it than to wait and later turn out to need it badly.

On the other hand, you wouldn't want to start treating for an active COVID-19 infection every time you sneeze or feel tired.

Please understand that in medicine there is often uncertainty at the beginning of an illness. But that uncertainty usually doesn't last. The illness declares itself quickly as time progresses. So if you are not sure, endure a few hours of watchful waiting. See how all the values are trending. In most cases, the way will soon be clear. Just don't let the watchful waiting drag on too long.

You might have the idea that medicine is an exact science. For the most part it is most definitely not. In clinic we make decisions based on probabilities more often than on certainties. For example, if a doctor sees someone in clinic for headache and there are no other red flags, they will probably diagnose a tension headache. That same headache could be a brain tumor or the beginning of an artery bleeding into the brain, but the chances are pretty low. It wouldn't be practical to get an MRI on everyone with a headache.

Time is of the essence in clinic, and one often does not want to wait for tests to come back before starting treatment. In the haze and confusion of the COVID-19 epidemic this is particularly true, especially since the tests are so questionable. So doctors often make a clinical diagnosis, which means, "We haven't proven it with tests yet, but this is what it looks like in clinic." Or they make a presumptive diagnosis, which means, "We don't have definite proof, but this is what it looks like at the moment, and we are going to act accordingly."

In the current epidemic, I would not rely on diagnostic tests at all. In my mind they simply cause delay and confusion. I have spent more than a few hours looking into the science of the PCR test and am convinced it is entirely misguided and unreliable. (Yet almost all of the statistics describing this epidemic are based on it.) As to the other tests, I have heard enough negative reports to put me off. Perhaps in the future testing will become more reliable and prompt. Delay for testing is not acceptable.

Gather All Your Data Points

In medicine, diagnosing is like looking at a pointilist

painting. You see a lot of dots. For a doctor, those dots are the pieces of information that they have. Your temperature is one dot. Your pulse oximeter reading is another dot. Each symptom is another dot. Then you stand back and see what image is formed by all those dots.

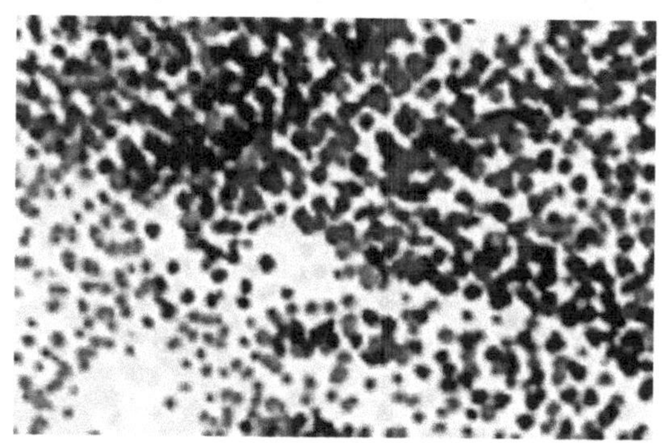

Above are some of the dots from the painting below. They don't make much sense until you stand back and look at all the dots.

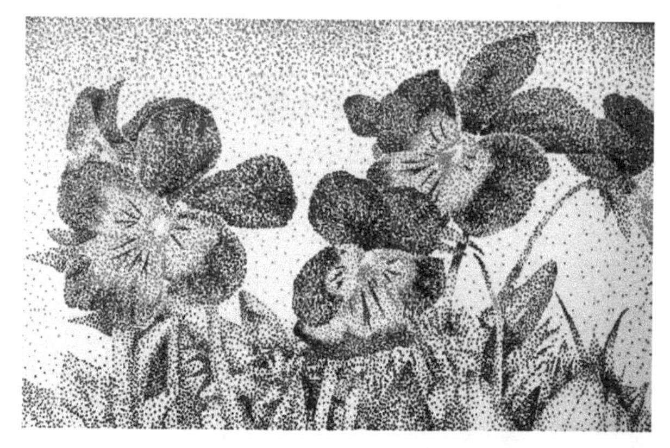

We are Interested in Signs and Symptoms

- Signs are what the healthcare person finds on examination. This would include pulse rate, what the lungs sound like through the stethoscope, blood pressure and so on.
- Symptoms are what the patient says they feel.

When it comes to numbers (such as heart rate, temperature, blood Oxygen saturation), we are very often more interested in changes and trends than in absolute values. There is no single, normal temperature or heart rate for humans. (There are, though, ranges outside of which a healthcare person would become concerned).

Since there are no absolute normals, I recommend you get a baseline of your vital signs while you are well. Then changes and trends will tell you very quickly when things are not going in the right direction.

What information would we gather to see if it's time to start the Ivermectin regimen?

1. How do I feel?

Many who suffer from COVID-19 (which, remember, is only a very small minority of people who get COVID-19) report feeling a kind of toxic, poisonous feeling they have never felt before. Don't ignore that feeling just because we can't measure it with a gizmo.

The three most common symptoms of COVID-19:

- Cough (57%)
- Fatigue (71%) and
- Loss of taste and/or smell (80%)

COVID-19 does sometimes have unusual symptoms:

- Loss of taste or smell
- "COVID-19 toes" - itchy, painful rashes on the fingers and toes

Other symptoms of COVID-19 are common for any cold or flu:

- headache
- muscle aches
- chills
- sore throat

- red, dry or itchy eyes
- nausea
- loss of appetite
- vomiting
- diarrhea
- shortness of breath (but see "silent hypoxia" below)
- rash

2. How do I look?

Have someone look at you, and go look in the mirror. Trust what is seen. My grandfather always said, "The patient knows what's wrong with them."

Vladimir Zelenko, MD was one of the first proponents of HCQ for COVID-19. He gave an interview in which he said that after he had treated over 4,000 COVID-19 patients, he could tell who had the illness just by looking at them.

3. What are my vital signs?

Vital signs are measurements you can take. They can help you tell when things are OK, when it's time to call in for healthcare advice, and when it's time to get to the Emergency Room or call 911.

Remember: vital signs are as much about trends as about specific numbers. You'll read, for example, that a normal temperature is 98.6°F. But that is really just the average temperature of the population. Many perfectly healthy people have temperatures slightly higher or lower than that. Be prepared – get some baseline valucs while you feel well. Keep a little notebook with your baseline values, and bring this notebook into play if you fall ill.

For COVID-19 the Key Vital Signs Are:

1. **Blood oxygen saturation.** In mild to moderate c, the blood oxygen saturation is still normal. In severe COVID-19 the blood oxygen saturation drops. (You take the blood oxygen saturation reading with a gizmo called a pulse oximeter. This shows what percentage of the blood in your arteries is carrying oxygen. (See **APPENDIX 4: Buying and Using the Pulse** Oximeter for more details.)
2. **Respiratory rate** (How many times you breathe in a minute)
3. **Temperature**
4. **Pulse** (how many times the heart beats per minute)

5. **Blood Pressure** (take this with a blood pressure cuff)

Silent Hypoxia: The Reason That Knowing the Blood Oxygen Saturation is Crucial

Of all the key vital signs, the Blood Oxygen Saturation is the most important. This is because COVID-19 has a quirk that all the other colds and flu don't have – **silent hypoxia.**

Fatigue is the mark of most viral colds and flu. It is one of the body's ways of telling you to lie low because there's healing to be done. Healing takes a lot of energy. (One of the main reasons many illnesses don't heal in our culture is because people simply can't or won't stop and rest.)

But in COVID-19, the fatigue can become incredibly severe for quite another reason – the lungs may not be getting enough oxygen into the blood. Normally when not enough oxygen is getting into the blood we feel short of breath. The body basically says, "Hey buddy, start breathing more! We're not getting enough oxygen!" With COVID-19 that shortness-of-breath message often doesn't get sent. This is unique to COVID-19.

When the oxygen level in the blood drops, that is a key red flag that tells you COVID-19 is getting serious. Watch out. And the only way you would know that is by having that little gizmo - the pulse oximeter. So it's well worthwhile to invest a little time and money in having and learning to use a pulse oximeter.

Do Things to Prevent Clotting

When COVID-19 is symptomatic, the immediate concern is that the body will so over-react to the infection that it induces the cytokine storm. One of the main risks of the cytokine storm is excess clotting of the blood.

Cytokines basically are chemical messengers in your body that tell your immune system to go into action. But remember that activation of the immune system goes hand-in-hand with inflammation. The cytokine storm is a form of extreme inflammation. With inflammation, the blood clots more easily. When the blood clots too much, blood flow is blocked and tissues don't receive the life-giving oxygen and nutrients they need. Therefore, when COVID-19 is symptomatic, the risk of blood clots increases. It is important to start doing things that would prevent the blood from clotting too easily.

Easy Ways to Prevent Blood Clots

1. Hydrate! You may feel terrible, and you might not be at all thirsty. You might feel as if you don't have the energy to get out of bed to fill your water bottle. Nonetheless, it is essential that you continually flush out your system by drinking enough fluids.

Dehydration will reliably make your blood more likely to clot. **Drink!**

How will you know if you are taking enough fluids? By the urine. If the urine is dark yellow, that is not good. It means you are concentrating your urine to preserve fluids. If the urine is light yellow or clear, you are getting in enough fluids.

(But note: some things can change the color of your urine. In that case, the light urine rule doesn't apply. A good example is a B Vitamin called Riboflavin.)

2. Move! The pumping of the heart is only part of the way that blood moves around the body. The contractions of our skeletal muscles help squeeze the blood along. I know it might seem like climbing Mount Everest just to get out of bed and do some gentle movement. Nevertheless, get up and do what you can to keep moving, even if it's only for a few minutes four or five times a day.

3. Breathe! When you take a deep breath, the blood is drawn back towards the heart from the periphery. This aids blood circulation. Stand up and take ten deep breaths four times a day.

4. Do Bed Yoga: Even if you can't get up out of bed, you can do gentle stretching where you lie. Each stretch squeezes blood out of the muscles and back toward the heart.

5. Keep the Bowels Open: When toxins accumulate, inflammation intensifies and the likelihood of clotting increases. The bowels are one important way by which we get rid of toxins. So do whatever it takes to keep the bowels open (fiber, magnesium, prunes, abdominal massage, senna, and so on).

6. Take Aspirin if it doesn't conflict with other medicines. Aspirin is the most common over-the-counter anti-coagulant. (An anti-coagulant is something that stops your blood from clotting so easily). The FLCCC recommends Aspirin 325 mg a day for early, out-patient COVID-19.

7. Consider natural foods, herbs and supplements which keep the blood moving. But please remember that, be it a chemical, a supplement or an herb, the only difference between a medicine and a poison is the dose. If you use too many blood thinning herbs you can bleed too easily, and that is a whole different and dangerous problem. Please use judgement and common sense. Don't overdo it. If you overreact out of fear and take excessively high doses, you are likely to make things worse.

Here are Some Herbs and Supplements that Thin the Blood

Turmeric: This herb is used in Chinese medicine to stimulate blood flow. It is commonly used in cooking and is usually available fresh in health food stores. You could also consider capsules of the active ingredient of tumeric, which is curcumin.

(See, for example, the article at http://www.bmbreports.org/journal/view.html?volume=45&number=4&spage=221)

Ginger: Ginger basically contains the same active ingredient as Aspirin *(salicylate),* but in milder form.

Cayenne: This herb is also quite rich in salicylates.

Cinnamon: Cinnamon contains Coumarin, a powerful blood-thinning agent. Coumadin, one of the most commonly used blood-thinning medications in Western medicine, is derived from Coumarin.

Nattokinase: Nattokinase is a natural enzyme derived from fermented soy beans. It is usually available where food supplements are sold. It decreases the blood's tendency to clot.

Should I Take Antibiotics if I Have Symptomatic COVID-19?

There is debate about this question. Mostly doctors now are saying no, don't take antibiotics unless there is some other specific reason. Earlier in the epidemic, they thought that part of the problem was that bacteria would come and infect the lungs, which were already weakened by the COVID-19 virus. But this is often not turning out to be true.

CHAPTER 7

Severe COVID-19

If COVID-19 progresses to severe, you should immediately either:

- Call your healthcare person—I would not wait more than an hour or two for them to call back. Instead I would proceed to the next steps.
- Go to the Emergency Room or
- Dial 911.

How Will I Know if COVID-19 is Becoming Serious?

There are two key signs that COVID-19 is going from mild or moderate to severe:

1. A drop in the blood oxygen saturation as measured by pulse oximeter.

   - They usually give as the alarm value **below 94%**, but this assumes normal values when you are well. It also assumes that you are near sea level. Get some baseline values in advance so you know when the values are dropping.

2. An increase in the number of breaths per minute. A normal breathing rate is considered, on average, to be 12-16 breaths/minute for adults. But this is one value for which you really want a baseline. For adults, if the breaths/minute goes over 27, it's definitely time for action. Do remember, though, many things can make one breath faster, include fear and fever.

Most other signs and symptoms of severe COVID-19 are basically a worsening of any or all of the symptoms of mild COVID-19.

Certain other serious signs demand immediate action:

- confusion
- sleepy and you can't rouse them
- so weak they can't move about

Clearly, then, it's advisable to have someone around to watch you (or at least check in regularly by phone) if you fall seriously ill from COVID-19.

Should I Start Taking Antibiotics if COVID-19 Worsens?

Current opinion elsewhere seems to be that we don't need antibiotics unless there is a specific reason.

Early in the epidemic, many healthcare people routinely gave antibiotics with the idea that since the lungs were impaired, the risk of bacteria coming to infect the lungs on top of the COVID-19 was high *(bacterial superinfection)*. Harvey Risch, MD and Vladimir Zelenko, MD still recommend antibiotics as part of the HCQ-based regimen, and the results are wonderful.

If you do feel antibiotics are needed, some have been using:

- Azithromycin 500 mg twice a day for five days. while others use:
- Doxycycline 200 mg followed by 100 mg daily for 5 days.

When COVID-19 Becomes Serious

A large percentage of COVID-19 infections are entirely without symptoms. Most COVID-19 infections with symptoms resolve on their own with a little rest and self-care. Only a very small percentage go on to become serious.

Many people with mild COVID-19 symptoms go to the Emergency Room. The policy of Emergency Rooms at the time of this writing is to send you home unless you are quite ill. It's kind of like calling the Fire Department and saying, "There is a fire in my kitchen," and having them reply, "Too bad. Call us when the whole house is on fire. Then we'll spring into action."

Therefore, it makes sense not to go to the Emergency Room for a mild COVID-19 infection. It would only stress you out, drain your energy, and potentially infect others.

On the other hand, seeking help promptly if things should start to go wrong is absolutely key. Time is of the essence when COVID-19 goes bad, and every hour counts.

It becomes crucial, then, to be able to recognize when to sound the alarm that COVID-19 is going in the wrong direction.

When COVID-19 becomes serious, the treatment changes. Additional medicines need to be brought into play. These medicines are:

- Something to stop the cytokine storm *(anti-inflammatory steroids)*
- Oxygen to breathe (*supplemental oxygen*)
- Something to keep your blood from clotting too easily *(anticoagulants)*

If you can get prompt treatment at an Emergency Room, they will know to start these medicines immediately. Some hospitals, I have heard, are even starting to use Ivermectin. But for the most part, these days, you are going to have to bring your own.

If, for whatever reason, you anticipate that there could be a delay in treatment, then you might want to have on hand some version of the three medicines above - anti-inflammatory steroids, anti-coagulants and supplemental oxygen.

In these times it's not hard to imagine that such a delay in treatment could occur. There have already been supply chain shortages for some medical supplies in this epidemic. There have already been instances where hospital Emergency Rooms were completely overwhelmed and there were long waits and delays in getting treatment. You might live in a remote area where it takes hours to get to the hospital. Or there could be road closures due to severe weather or due to civil unrest. There could be other collapses of infrastructure, such as a gas shortages.

The focus of this section of the manual is to give you the skills to know when it's time to go to the next level of treatment and call in the healthcare system.

However, if you do decide you want to be ready for any eventuality, I have included some appendices that give you a starting point:

- **APPENDIX 5: Anti-inflammatory Steroids for COVID-19**
- **APPENDIX 6: Home Oxygen for Severe COVID-19**
- **APPENDIX 7: Blood thinners (Anticoagulants) to Prevent Clotting in Severe COVID-19**

But please be clear: if you are going to have ready and know how to use these types of medicines for severe COVID-19, you will need more medical knowledge than this manual provides. I can only offer a point of departure.

Why the Treatment Changes When COVID-19 Becomes Severe

We currently think that, on average, the first five or so days of a COVID-19 infection there are few or no symptoms. The virus is replicating and the body is gearing up to fight the infection.

Then, sometime around day five, flu-like symptoms begin. Over the next seven days, more or less, the body quickly controls the infection and kills the virus.

However, after that seven days the body's immune system can become extremely overactivated and start attacking everything in sight, especially in the lungs. This is the cytokine storm, which is potentially fatal.

It's important to understand that the cytokine storm is not an active infection. It is the body's overreaction to the COVID-19 infection which has just been conquered.

Modern medicine has a very effective tool for tamping down the immune system frenzy which is the cytokine storm – anti-inflammatory steroids. Anti-inflammatory steroids cool out the entire immune system. But the timing of when to start use these steroids has to be right.

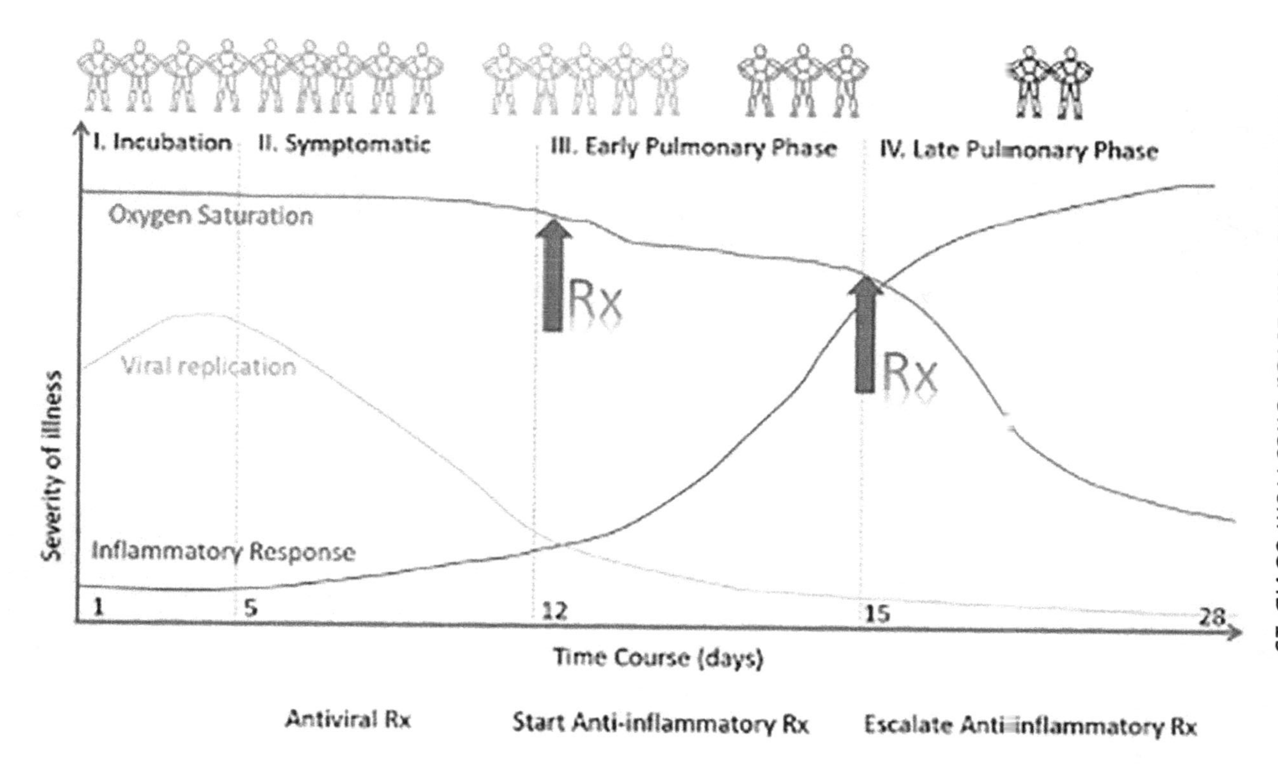
I. Incubation
II. Symptomatic
III. Early Pulmonary Phase
IV. Late Pulmonary Phase
Oxygen Saturation
Rx
Rx
Viral replication
Inflammatory Response
Severity of illness
1
5
12
15
28
Time Course (days)
Antiviral Rx
Start Anti-inflammatory Rx
Escalate Anti-inflammatory Rx

Timing is crucial in the use of anti-inflammatory steroids for COVID-19.

1. If you start steroids too soon, while the virus is still active, you interfere with the immune system's response in stopping the virus.

2. If you start steroids too late, it is like letting a runaway train gather momentum. The cytokine storm is much easier to nip in the bud than when it's in full bloom. So once the viral infection is more or less over and the cytokine storm is beginning, it's important to start steroids right away.

GRATITUDE

We are all fully interconnected, and we are all fully interconnected with the entire web of life on Earth. I feel that each one of us has to take responsibility, learn and actively cultivate our own health and the health of our family. I hope my work assists in that process.

If this manual saves one life, I will consider all the work and struggles of my medical career well-rewarded.

Please, if your spirit moves you, share this manual with your loved ones and with anyone you feel could receive its benefit. We all need to speak out until the truth is clear.

With a wish that all be healthy and happy,

Michael Arnold, MD, L.Ac.
18 April, 2021
Aptos, California

ACKNOWLEDGMENTS

I am grateful to everyone who helped bring this work to you. It definitely takes a tribe to write a book. It would not have been possible without all of you. Thank you!

I would especially like to thank:

Marlies Myoku Cocheret de La Morinière

For firm encouragement and spiritual guidance.

http://marliescocheret.com/

Mark Howard, M.D.

For sharing his expertise and extensive Emergency Room experience.

Dr. L. Francesca Ferrari, L.Ac.

For sharing both her clinical experience and her extensive research on the subject.

http://www.francescaferrari.com/

Frances Anagnost Williams, M.D.

For her spirited commitment to the truth, and for sharing her extensive clinical experience.

https://franceswilliamsmd.com/

Patricia Hamilton

For being my guide in the publishing wilderness, and for putting this book into form.
parkplacepublications.com

Ann Thompson, Ph.D.

For alerting me to Ivermectin in the first place, for her extensive information gathering, and for help with the proofreading.

Allan & Sun Lundell (Dr. & Mrs. Future)

For inviting me to publicly call it the way I saw it.
http://www.drfutureshow.com/

Julie Rybinski, RPh

For sharing her expertise as a Pharmacist, and for proofreading.

Pernilla Lillarose

For all the information she has sent, and for the bright light she shines.

Katia Wilder, PA, BS

For sharing both her extensive clinical experience and her knowledge.

John Lumiere-Wins

For a vast river of informational items.

The Covid Preparedness Workgroup

For caring and showing up.

Everyone in the Palace of Health

For encouraging me in my teaching about how to stay healthy.

The Skypad

For being a bubble of sanity in these crazy weird times.

Shyamala White

For her proofreading and enthusiasm.

APPENDICES

APPENDIX 1

Making Friends with Ivermectin

Ivermectin is a relatively safe and inexpensive medicine. There is a growing body of literature showing that Ivermectin is useful in the treatment of COVID-19. If you are going to take Ivermectin while not under the care of a medical doctor (and of course I, as a medical doctor, would never recommend this. I would probably lose my license if I did), it is important you be familiar with its side effects and drug interactions.

A Little Background on Ivermectin

In 2015, William C. Campbell and Satoshi Omura, the scientists who developed Ivermectin, won The Nobel Prize in Physiology or Medicine for their research.

Ivermectin was discovered in 1975 in Japan. It is processed from a chemical that is isolated from one specific kind of bacteria. In the United States, it is given to humans only by a doctor's prescription. In veterinary medicine, it is over-the-counter without a prescription for horses and some other animals.

Ivermectin was first used to treat parasites, including:

1. River blindness (Onchocerciasis) - this is the second most common cause of blindness from infection in the world. It occurs in tropical climates, when flies carrying the parasite bite humans.

2. Scabies - a disease in humans where the scabies mite burrows under the skin, causing intense itching.

3. Filariasis - a tropical disease where these worms block up the lymph vessel, causing huge swell-ings, especially in the legs.

4. Strongyloidiasis - a tropical disease caused by roundworms which burrow up through the soles of the feet into the body when people go barc-foot in infested areas.

How long does Ivermectin last in your Blood?

After you take Ivermectin, it reaches the highest concentration in the blood after between 31 and 47 hours. The half life is 18 hours. This means that every 18 hours the concentration of Ivermectin in a person's blood drops by half.

Ivermectin Dosage

The usual dose of Ivermectin for an adult of average size is 12 mg (milligrams) per dose).

Should you want to be more precise, doses are often given by body weight. The usual dose of Ivermectin is

Ivermectin 0.2 mg/kg

If you want to do the same calculation based on your body weight in pounds, it would be approximately:

Ivermectin 0.1 mg/lb (milligrams/pound)
(The exact number if 0.091 mg/lb)

So, as an example, the precise dose for a 100 pound person would be 9 mg. If, God forbid, you found yourself in a situation where you needed to take Ivermectin without consulting a physician, it would be very useful to be able to do this little bit of math.

Ivermectin Cautions and Contraindications

Ivermectin is a very safe medicine which has been taken very widely all over the world. Most people can take Ivermectin without any problem. But some medical conditions make it a little more dicey. They would include:

Liver disease: Ivermectin is processed in the liver and excreted through the bowels.

Kidney disease.

Ivermectin Side Effects

If you get side effects, stop taking the medication. In the very unlikely event that side effects become severe, contact your physician or go to the Emergency Room.

Of course, it's often not so simple to sort out side effects from the illness and other factors. For example, Ivermectin can, rarely, cause dizziness. But maybe you were just too sick to drink enough fluids and you feel dizzy because you're dehydrated. Or maybe you are one of the 2.8% who feel dizzy from the viral infection itself. It gets to be a judgement call.

In any case, here are the common side effects, and how often they occur:

General

exhaustion/fatigue (0.9%),

Digestive

abdominal pain (0.9%)
loss of appetite, can't eat (0.9%),
constipation (0.9%),
diarrhea (1.8%),
nausea (1.8%),
vomiting (0.9%),

Nervous System

dizziness (2.8%),
somnolence (0.9%),
vertigo (0.9%),
tremor (0.9%),

Skin

itching (2.8%),
rash (0.9%),
hives (0.9%).

Ivermectin Drug Interactions

While generally safe, Ivermectin does interact with a lot of things, especially medications. If you are going to take Ivermectin you should know what other medications you are on and whether or not they will interact.

Please note that Ivermectin does interact with **alcohol**. Alcohol changes the levels of Ivermectin in the blood.

Also please note that Ivermectin interacts with an herb called **Echinacea**.

On the next page is a list of medicines with which Ivermectin may interact. Please be aware that in modern medicine most medications have two names - a brand name and a generic name. This list gives the generic names. To use it, you should know the generic names of any medications you are taking. (For example, Valium is a brand name. The generic same for that same pill is "Diazepam.")

Ivermectin Drug Interactions

(From Drugs.comSearch)

- 70 moderate drug interactions
- 2 minor drug interactions

Medications known to interact with Ivermectin

Note: Showing generic names only.

A

Abametapir Topical

Amprenavir

Anisindione

Apalutamide

Aprepitant

Armodafinil

Atazanavir

B

Boceprevir

Bosentan

Brigatinib

C

Chloramphenicol

Clarithromycin

Cobicistat

Conivaptan

D

Darunavir

Dasatinib

Deferasirox

Delavirdine

Dicumarol

Dronedarone

Duvelisib

E

Efavirenz
Enzalutamide
Erythromycin
Ethanol
Etravirine

F

Fosamprenavir
Fosaprepitant
Fostamatinib

I

Idelalisib
Indinavir
Isavuconazonium
Itraconazole
Ivacaftor

K

Ketoconazole

L

Lapatinib
Larotrectinib
Lefamulin
Letermovir
Lorlatinib

M

Mibefradil
Mifepristone
Modafinil

N

Nefazodone
Nelfinavir
Nevirapine
Nilotinib

O

Oxcarbazepine

P

Pitolisant
Posaconazole

R

Ribociclib
Rifapentine
Ritonavir
Rucaparib
Rufinamide

S

Saquinavir
Selpercatinib
Sirolimus
Sodium Iodide I-123
Sodium Iodide-I-131
Somapacitan-Beco
Somatrem
Somatropin
Stiripentol

T

Tacrolimus
Telaprevir
Telithromycin
Telotristat
Temsirolimus
Troleandomycin
Tucatinib

V

Voriconazole

W

Warfarin

A Note About Ivermectin From a Friend Who Is a Physician

I have a friend who is a physician back east who uses Ivermectin for himself and his patients regularly. I asked him about his experience, and he had this to say:

"I am very casual on using Ivermectin myself. Ivermectin has been OTC ["Over-The-Counter"] in much of the world, including South America, Central America, and Africa. Anywhere that malaria and parasites are found. Tens of millions of doses have been distributed by Merck for river blindness parasites. I consider it an exceptionally safe drug for occasional use.

Escalating dose studies in humans show no adverse effects when 10x the standard dose (2 mg/Kg) is used. In farm animals, it is at about 50x the standard dose (10 mg/Kg) that they begin to get wobbly, have trouble walking and become uncoordinated. It is at 75x (15 mg/Kg) that they become comatose. There are several breeds of dogs that are MORE sensitive to Ivermectin than average (including collies), so in dogs caution is used. Keeping Ivermectin out of the brain depends on an intact blood brain barrier. So, it is ***possible*** that encephalitis/meningitis might reduce the safety margin of Ivm by damaging the Blood Brain-Barrier. Ivermectin is a GABA synapse neurotoxin, whose safety in humans is due to the blood brain barrier preventing brain access.

"No doctor, vet or pharmacist can EVER say that veterinary Ivermectin is safe for human use because application for human use of the horse paste (for example) has never been applied for, tested by the FDA or approved. So, nobody can ever publicly say it is OK. However, confidentially, several vets and a group of farmers have let me know that they personally use vet drugs and give them to family members and recommend them to close neighbors. A friend who is a large animal vet and farmer in the North East gives his entire family veterinary Ivermectin every 10 days through the winter to prevent COVID-19. For me personally, that is good enough. But for many it will not be. Such is the nature of the information warfare that we find going on around us. 'Tis sad and some will be lost because of this."

APPENDIX 2

Obtaining Ivermectin

1. Ivermectin by Prescription

In the United States, Ivermectin is given only by prescription. At this time it may not be so easy to find a physician willing to prescribe Ivermectin. If you have a doctor who is open-minded but not yet on board, it might be worthwhile to download and print out "Review of the Emerging Evidence Demonstrating the Efficacy of Ivermectin in the Prophylaxis and Treatment of COVID-19" from:

http://covid19criticalcare.com/wp-content/uploads/2020/11/FLCCC-Ivermectin-in-the-prophylaxis-and-treatment-of-COVID-19.pdf

Hand it to your doctor. Ask them to review the evidence.

It may help your physician to note that on January 14th, 2021 the National Institutes of Health (NIH) changed its stance on using Ivermectin for COVID-19. They are now "neither for nor against." This is the same status they currently give to monoclonal antibodies (like Regeneron)

and convalescent plasma – treatments about which few doctors have reservations.

Is it Legal in Your State for a Physician to Prescribe Ivermectin for COVID-19?

At this time the laws and standards in various states are in flux. I have not found a good summary of the situation. If you should happen upon one, please let me know.

Unfortunately, your doctors might not know if they are allowed to prescribe Ivermectin. I have heard more than one doctor refuse to prescribe Ivermectin because, "It might get me in trouble with the Medical Board," although they have no knowledge of that one way or the other, and apparently little inclination to find out.

I asked several friends to inquire of the Medical Board in my state if it were legal for a doctor to prescribe Ivermectin to have on hand in case of COVID-19 infection. More than six weeks later, neither of the inquiries have been answered.

2. Lists of Doctors Known to Prescribe Ivermectin for COVID-19

While I can make no warrantee or guarantee about the doctors on the lists below, here are some places to start looking.

A. This list is on the FLCCC website and includes doctors the world over:

https://COVID-1919criticalcare.com/network-support/the-flccc-alliance/

They also have a shorter list of US physicians here: https://covid19criticalcare.com/guide-for-this-website/take-action-and-share-the-infos-with-your-doctor/

B. This list is from a private group of concerned citizens:

https://www.exstnc.com/

C. This site connects you with a doctor for telemedicine:

https://speakwithanmd.com americasfrontlinedoctors/

D. Foreign Sources:

Ivermectin is inexpensive and over-the-counter in many other countries, including Mexico, Argentina, and Iraq.

E. Other Sources of Ivermectin

As the medical system is limiting peoples' access to Ivermectin, some have resorted to taking veterinary Ivermectin made for horses. This is available over-the-counter in most pet stores in the USA. While the CDC and the FDA strongly recommend against this, I could find no specific reason that would make the veterinary preparation for horses toxic or otherwise unsuitable for humans.

You might, God forbid, find yourself in a situation where your choice was veterinary Ivermectin or no Ivermectin. You might find yourself in a situation where you felt it was very important to take Ivermectin. Sort of a wilderness medicine situation. If you are in a pinch and decide to take veterinary Ivermectin, please read the label carefully for other ingredients.

As it turns out, I have reports that taking horse Ivermectin simplifies the dosing issue. The dose for horses by weight is the same as the dose for humans. Horse Ivermectin comes with a syringe with gradations marked by weight. So if you must, just pretend you're a filly and don't overdo it.

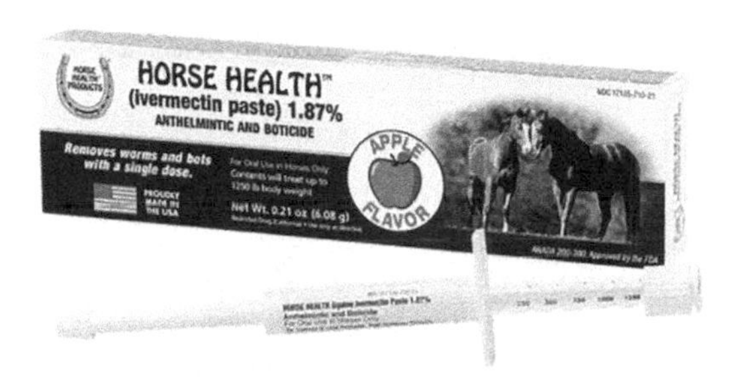

You will find dire warnings on the veterinary Ivermectin label that it is not for humans, but I know more than a few humans who have taken it without ill consequence. Examining the label and searching on the web, I could find nothing that would suggest a human would have problems taking veterinary Ivermectin (beyond a vague warning from the FDA).

APPENDIX 3

Knowledgeable Experts

In the vast tsunami of confusion flying around the digital world these days it's easy to get overwhelmed. They call it analysis paralysis. How do you sort out the truth?

I've developed a few simple guidelines:

1. Consider the source. Are they knowledgeable experts? If someone doesn't even give their name, it's not worth listening to what they have to say.

2. Have they looked into the matter, or are they just repeating something they heard because it sounded true to them? Personally, I have spent hundreds, if not thousands, of hours looking into the science of the COVID-19 situation before arriving at my opinions on the matter.

3. What do they have to gain or lose? Follow the money. The reason the scientific literature has become unreliable is that it takes huge amounts of money to do the kind of research that is considered legitimate these days. The money controls the results.

Considerations of power, career advancement and status have supplanted the truth as a top priority.

4. Go check what they say. If they cite a certain article, go look it up and see if it actually says what they are saying that it says. You would be surprised how often it is not.

5. Consider the tone. Is it reasoned and calm, or angry, judgmental and alarmist?

6. The more someone considers their opinion as established fact and absolute truth, the less I trust their opinion.

7. Points off for music. Programmatic music tells you what to feel. No thank you. Just give me the information and I will decide what I feel about it.

In my research into Ivermectin, I have relied on the views of highly qualified, knowledgeable experts. By listening to them and checking what they say, I have come to trust them. These experts have decades of training and experience in their fields. When I listen to them, they make sense. When I follow up on their sources, they are confirmed.

Zack Bush, MD
https://zachbushmd.com/

- MD, University of Colorado Health Sciences Center, May 2001
- Residency in Internal Medicine, University of Virginia Health System, 2002 – 2005
- Fellowship in Endocrinology/Metabolism, University of Virginia Health System, 2006 – 2009
- Internship in Hospice/Palliative Care at Hospice of the Piedmont, 2010 – 2014

Of all the perspectives I have studied on the COVID-19 epidemic and our response to it, the views of Dr. Bush have been the most informed and profound. It is a joy to listen to him talk about the web of life and how we, as living beings fit into it. I would definitely start here if I were to go further.

Here's a good podcast to start with:

file:///Zach Bush - Our COVID-19 Assumptions Are Wrong/ Why Social Distancing & Vaccines Will Make This Pandemic Worse

Andrew Kaufman, MD
https://andrewkaufmanmd.com/

- MD from Medical University of South Carolina
- BS in Molecular Biology from MIT
- Board Certified in Psychiatry after training at Duke University Medical Center

Dr. Kaufman challenges the science behind the COVID-19 epidemic. He also challenges the validity of the PCR test. He scientifically describes the flaws in our approach to the coronavirus.

James Lyons-Weiler, Ph.D.
https://jameslyonsweiler.com/

- B.S. in Zoology and Paleoecology from Ohio State University
- Ph.D. in Ecology, Evolution, and Conservation Biology
- Postdoctoral degree in Computational Molecular Biology at Penn State University

Describes the issues of Pathogenic Priming and Antibody Dependent Enhancement which have stopped the attempts to develop a vaccine against coronaviruses in the past (SARS and MERS).

Here's a good interview by him:
https://www.bitchute.com/video/NOzpwzTsMayS/

Paul E. Marik, MD, FCCM, FCCP

https://COVID-1919criticalcare.com/wp-content/uploads/2021/01/FLCCC-Alliance-member-CV-Marik.pdf

- MBBCh, Bachelor of Medicine and Surgery, University of Witwaterstrand
- D.Hom.Med, Diploma in Alternative Medicine, Bantridge Forest School, Sussex, UK
- D.Av.Med, Diploma in Aviation Medicine, South African Defense Force
- M.Med, Master of Medicine, University of Witwaterstrand
- BSc (Hons) Pharmacology, University of Witwaterstrand
- DTM&H, Diploma in Tropical Medicine and Hygiene, University of Witwaterstrand
- FCP (SA), College of Medicine of South Africa
- DA (DA), Diploma of Anesthesia, College of Medicine of South Africa
- FRCPC, Royal College of Physicians and Surgeons of Canada

- PNS, American Board of Physician Nutrition Specialists
- UCNS–NCC, United Council for Neurological Subspecialities
- South African Medical and Dental Council, General Practitioner, Specialty certification in Internal Medicine, Sub-specialty certification in Critical Care Medicine
- British Medical Council, General Practitioner, Specialty certification in Internal Medicine
- Canadian Medical Council, General Practitioner, Specialty certification in Internal Medicine, Sub-specialty certification in Critical Care Medicine
- American Board of Internal Medicine (ABIM), Internal Medicine, Critical Care Medicine
- American Board of Physician Nutrition Specialists, Physician Nutrition Specialist
- United Council for Neurological Subspecialities (USA), Neurocritical Care Specialist

One of the founders of the FLCCC.

Pierre Kory, MD

https://COVID-1919criticalcare.com/wp-content/uploads/2021/01/FLCCC-Alliance-member-CV-Kory.pdf

- 1988–1994 B.A. University of Colorado, Boulder, Colorado Major Mathematics
- 1994–1996 M.P.A. New York University, New York, NY Health Policy and Administration
- 1998–2002 MD St. George's University Grenada, West Indies
- 2002–2005 Residency Internal Medicine, Columbia College of Physicians and Surgeons, New York, NY, St. Luke's–Roosevelt Hospital, New York
- 2005–2008 Fellowship Pulmonary Disease and Critical Care Medicine Albert Einstein College of Medicine, Beth Israel Medical Center, New York
- Certification
    - Board Certified in Internal Medicine
    - Board Certified in Pulmonary Diseases
    - Board Certified in Critical Care Medicine

One of the founders of the FLCCC.

Harvey Risch, MD
https://medicine.yale.edu/profile/harvey_risch/?tab=bio

- Professor of Epidemiology in the Department of Epidemiology and Public Health at the Yale School of Public Health and Yale School of Medicine
- Postdoctoral Fellow in Epidemiology, School of Public Health and Community Medicine, University of Washington (1983)
- Ph.D., University of Chicago (1980)
- MD, University of California, San Diego (1976)
- B.S., California Institute of Technology (1972)
- Associate Editor of the *Journal of the National Cancer Institute*
- Editor of the *International Journal of Cancer*
- Was for six years a Member of the Board of Editors, the *American Journal of Epidemiology*

Dr. Risch was one of the first voices insisting that there were already FDA-approved medicines that could effectively be re-purposed for the early treatment of COVID-19. He has stood firm in the storm that followed.

Here is an extract of his courageous testimony on the subject before the US Senate:

https://www.youtube.com/watch?v=R4HTsgHAlUY

Vladimir Zelenko, MD

https://vladimirzelenkomd.com/

- MD, State University of New York, Buffalo, NY, 2000.
- Family Medicine residency, South Nassau Communities Hospital, 2004
- BA, Summa Cum Laude, Chemistry, Hofstra University

Dr. Zelenko stood in clinic fearlessly when his Long Island, NY community was one of the areas that was hardest hit by COVID-19. His HCQ approach has succeeded with thousands of patients.

Here is an interview about his experience:

https://covexit.com/dr-zelenko-interview-part-1/

Geert Vanden Bossche, DVM, PhD
https://www.geertvandenbossche.org/

- DVM from the University of Ghent, Belgium.
- PhD in Virology, University of Hohenheim, Germany.
- Has worked for several vaccine companies (GSK Biologicals, Novartis Vaccines, Solvay Biologicals.)
- Has worked in vaccine R&D.
- Has worked for the Bill & Melinda Gates Foundation's Global Health Discovery team in Seattle (USA) as Senior Program Officer.
- Has worked for the Global Alliance for Vaccines and Immunization (GAVI) in Geneva as Senior Ebola Program Manager.
- Has worked at the German Center for Infection Research in Cologne as Head of the Vaccine Development Office.
- Served as a Biotech/Vaccine consultant while also conducting his own research on Natural Killer cell-based vaccines.

- Here is a link to his full CV:

https://37b32f5a-6ed9-4d6d-b3e1-5ec648ad9ed9.filesusr.com/ugd/28d8fe_9bb701b3fd734d7895bc9b502752684f.pdf

Dr. Vanden Bossche's concerns are more regarding the vaccines than regarding Ivermectin. In the last couple of months Dr. Vanden Bossche, a mainstream vaccine advocate if there ever was one, shocked the world by saying that vaccines given during an active epidemic are only going to select for more powerful mutations. Thus, he says, this approach is only going to make matters worse.

https://www.youtube.com/watch?v=mUIDeCRDLnU&t=19s

Kary Mullis, Ph.D.
https://www.karymullis.com/

- BS, 1966, Georgia Institute of Technology
  PhD, 1973, University of California, Berkeley
- Nobel Prize in Chemistry, 1993 for developing the PCR test

Kary Mullis invented the test used to justify the idea that there is a COVID-19 epidemic – the PCR test. He was adamant that his test could not be used for the diagnosis of any disease. PCR is a research test to be used in the laboratories. It is not a clinical test.

Kary Mullis explains why his PCR test is not a diagnostic test:

https://www.youtube.com/watch?v=rXm9kAhNj-4

https://www.reddit.com/r/NoNewNormal/comments/kdtssx/the_creator_of_the_pcr_test_dr_kary_mullis/

Mobeen Syed, MD
https://www.drbeen.com/team/

- MD, 2004, King Edward University

Dr. Been is a medical educator and a strong advocate of Ivermectin.

He has many educational videos on COVID-19, Ivermectin and other subjects at:

https://www.youtube.com/c/USMLEOnline/playlists

Ryan Cole, MD

https://independentdocsid.com/RyanColeMD

- MD, 1997, Virginia Commonwealth University School of Medicine
- Board-certified dermatopathologist
- CEO/Medical Director of Cole Diagnostics.
- Dermatopathology Fellowship (Chief Fellow). Mayo Clinic (July 1997-June 2002)
- Resident in Anatomic and Clinical Pathology. Chief Fellow,
- Surgical Pathology Fellowship. Medical College of Virginia (1993-1997): Researched immunology.

https://www.bitchute.com/video/nAWbvsCBM2JG/

Here Dr. Cole gives a clear, practical view of the current status of the COVID-19 epidemic:

- "We are out of the pandemic."
- "You cannot get the cytokine storm if you have a normal Vitamin D level."
- "If you are obese, you are inflamed." And inflammation predisposes to the cytokine storm.

John Ioannides, MD

https://profiles.stanford.edu/john-ioannidis

- MD, University of Athens, 1990
- Residency: Internal Medicine, Harvard Medical School
- Fellowship: Infectious Diseases, Tufts University School of Medicine
- Ph.D. in Epidemiology and Clinical Research, Stanford University
- Professor of Medicine and Director, Stanford Prevention Research Center, Stanford University School of Medicine
- Professor of Biomedical Data Science, Stanford University School of Medicine

John Ioannidis, MD, Ph.D. is an incredibly qualified scientist and researcher. Yet he has concluded that you can't trust the scientific literature anymore. Too much of it is exaggerated, misleading or flat-out false. These days we often see people thumping their hand on a stack of scientific papers, asserting, "These are the FACTS!" Don't believe them. Many researchers publish what suits their employers, what will further their careers, or what will get them the next infusion of grant money.

For a simple first pass at his point of view, read, "*Lies, Damn Lies and Medical Science*" (The Atlantic, November, 2010)

https://www.theatlantic.com/magazine/archive/2010/11/lies-damned-lies-and-medical-science/308269/)

Here he discusses how the lockdown was not good medicine:

https://www.youtube.com/watch?v=cwPqmLoZA4s

APPENDIX 4

Buying and Using a Pulse Oximeter

Say what now? A pulse oxy what-the-what?

We need to know when you're not getting enough oxygen out of the air and into your blood. The pulse oximeter measures how much oxygen is getting into the blood. In COVID-19, if the amount of oxygen getting into the blood drops, that is a sure sign the problem has gone to the lungs and the cytokine storm is underway. Immediate action is crucial.

"Pulse Oximeter" is just short for "Pulse Oxygen Meter." It's a meter that looks at the blood in your pulse to see how much oxygen is getting into your blood. You just clip the sensor onto your finger, turn on the gizmo and away it goes. Easy and painless.

Why is a pulse oximeter essential in the COVID-19 epidemic?

Over 99% of COVID-19 infections have only mild or no symptoms. Rarely, COVID-19 goes badly, affects the lungs, and incites a storm of inflammation called the cytokine storm.

In the rare cases when COVID-19 goes bad, there is often an unusual feature: the person doesn't feel short of breath, but when you check the amount of oxygen in the blood, it is quite low. They call this situation **silent hypoxia**, which simply means "silent low oxygen in the blood."

In any illness, you always have to look at the whole picture. You can't just focus in on one sign or symptom. That being said, a low level of oxygen in the blood is a major red flag that COVID-19 has gone beyond an annoying viral infection and has become life-threatening. The pulse oximeter is key to knowing if and when it's time to head for the Emergency Room.

If the level of oxygen in the blood does fall, success in treatment depends on starting treatment immediately (with oxygen, anti-inflammatory steroids such as methylprednisolone, and blood thinners).

Buying a Pulse Oximeter

A pulse oximeter is kind of like a seatbelt or a smoke alarm. You hope you never need it. But if you do end up needing it, you surely want one that is good and reliable.

So which pulse oximeter should you buy?

The most reliable pulse oximeters are approved by the FDA for medical use. They are only available with a doctor's prescription, and they are quite expensive.

The other class of pulse oximeters are designated "not for medical use" (NMU). They are much less expensive, and they will do quite nicely for our purposes. This is because we really only need to know if the oxygen in the blood drops below a certain point *(Authors are putting that somewhere around 93% these days)*. At a value of 90% or above, the inexpensive, NMU pulse oximeters are relatively reliable.

The consensus is, though, that it's the trend of the pulse oximeter values that matter. So take a bunch of readings while you are well. If you fall ill, take a few readings every day and note the values.

Here are some tips for buying a pulse oximeter that my research has suggested so far:

1. Get a stand-alone pulse oximeter that works on your fingers. The ones that work through smart phones are not as reliable.

2. Get a pulse oximeter that also tells you the strength of the pulse signal. This is a measure of how clearly the pulse oximeter sees the blood in your arteries.

Why? The blood in your arteries moves in squirts. The blood in your veins has more of an oozing motion. The blood in the arteries has lots of oxygen. The blood in the veins has much less oxygen. We are interested in seeing how much oxygen is in the arteries, not the veins. To tell the blood in the arteries from the blood in the veins the pulse ox needs to clearly see the squirts of blood in the arteries. Pulse signal tells you how clearly the pulse ox is seeing those squirts.

As far as specific brands, it's hard to tell. Without endorsing any specific product or website, this website sounded credible:

https://nursefocus.net/7-BEST-PULSE-OXIMETERS-REVIEWS-BUYERS-GUIDE/

Here are a couple of links with more general comments about pulse oximeters:

Consumer Reports

https://www.consumerreports.org/medical-symptoms/COVID-19-pulse-oximeters-oxygen-levels-faq/

FDA

https://www.fda.gov/consumers/consumer-updates/pulse-oximeters-and-oxygen-concentrators-what-know-about-home-oxygen-therapy

It's important to be aware that pulse oximeters were basically developed for white people. They are somewhat less accurate in darker skinned people. (for more details see "Racial Bias in Pulse Oximetry Measurement" https://www.nejm.org/doi/pdf/10.1056/NEJMc2029240?articleTools=true)

How to Use Your Pulse Oximeter

These suggestions apply to the kind of pulse oximeter you clip on your finger.

1. Get some baseline values while you are healthy.

   The trend of the readings is far more important than the individual readings. This is especially true since not all pulse oximeters are extremely accurate.

2. Tips for getting good readings:

- If you have some illness wherein your baseline oxygen is less than 90%, the over-the-counter pulse oximeters will be less accurate. You might want to obtain a FDA approved medical-use pulse oximeter via a doctor's prescription.
- Pulse oximeters were developed for white people. They are somewhat less accurate in darker skinned people. (for more details: Racial Bias in Pulse Oximetry Measurement https://www.nejm.org/doi/pdf/10.1056/NEJMc2029240?articleTools=true)
- Remove any nail polish.
- Use the index or middle finger for the reading.

- Take the reading at rest and not just after exertion.
- The pulse oximeter needs to see a good pulse. If there is not a good pulse, then just know the reading may be less accurate. That is why it is good to have a device that also tells you the strength of the pulse signal. Things that might interfere with a good pulse are blockages in the arteries of the arms (from diseases like diabetes or heart disease), low blood pressure, and medicines such as albuterol which make the arteries tighten down.
- If you are very overweight, take the reading while sitting up straight. Lying down or hunching forward may limit how much the lungs can fill up with air. This could give a low reading which has nothing to do with COVID-19 in the lungs.
- Make measurements indoors, at rest.
- Take the measurement after breathing quietly and not talking for a few minutes.
- Watch the reading for about a minute. It may jump around. Take a value in the middle of what you see.

- If the fingers are cold, warm them up before trying to take the measurement.
- If ill, take readings two or three times daily and keep a log recording the values. The trend is the key issue.
- Be aware that at higher altitudes, the oxygen saturation may be lower just because there's less oxygen in the air.
- Remember that COVID-19 is not the only reason someone's oxygen saturation could drop. But if you have COVID-19 and the oxygen saturation drops, COVID-19 is certainly the most likely reason.

APPENDIX 5

Anti-inflammatory Steroids for Severe COVID-19

Methylprednisolone adult dose:

- 80 mg to start,
- Then 40 mg every 12 hours for a minimum of 7 days.
- Evidence shows that if you stop before 7 days, the cytokine storm may come back.
- When stopping anti-inflammatory steroids, it is better to taper off slowly than to stop suddenly.

OR

Prednisone:

- 100 mg to start,
- Then 50 mg every 12 hours for at least 7 days.
- Evidence shows that if you stop before 7 days, the cytokine storm may come back. When stopping anti-inflammatory steroids, it is better to taper off slowly than to stop suddenly.

Do not take both Methylprednisolone and Prednisone at once. That would be an overdose.

Methylprednisolone seems to be a little better than Prednisone for severe COVID-19, but Prednisone is more commonly available.

How Anti-Inflammatory Steroids Work

With COVID-19, it's the cytokine storm that's the problem. The body controls the virus, no problem. But the immune system can be thrown so out of whack that the immune over-reaction can actually go on to kill the body.

When the cytokine storm is threatening, we want a medicine that will turn down the intensity of the immune system. We have such medicines in a class called anti-inflammatory steroids. These are medicines against inflammation. Some examples are Prednisone, Dexamethasone and Methylprednisolone. People commonly take them for things like asthma, auto-immune diseases and poison oak.

Please don't confuse this type of steroid with other types of steroids. You hear about sex hormones, which are a type of steroid, and also about the anabolic steroids which athletes and weightlifters may abuse. Anti-inflammatory steroids are quite different. They just lower the intensity with which the immune system is acting. It's like Valium for your white blood cells.

Timing is key when using anti-inflammatory steroids. You don't want to tamp down the immune system while it's dealing with the virus. But when the virus is defunct and the immune system is spinning out of control, you want to tamp down the immune system on the spot.

The general model now is that with a COVID-19 infection there is first a period where the person is infected, but there are no symptoms yet. This lasts an average of five days.

Then the symptoms showing that the body is fighting the virus appear – fever, fatigue and so on. This lasts on average about a week.

Usually after that week of symptoms there is a slow recovery and return to normal. But for a very few, there is a turning point for the worse. The cytokine storm begins to kick in. It is at exactly at this point in time that one should start anti-inflammatory steroids (as well as oxygen and anti-coagulants).

If you start anti-inflammatory steroids too soon, it can interfere with the body's ability to conquer the virus. If you start them too late, it is like waiting to call the Fire Department when your house is on fire. This is why following the breathing rate and the blood oxygen saturation is so key. When the cytokine storm starts, it begins to interfere with lung function and that shows up when measuring those values.

Anti-inflammatory steroids are powerful medicines with potentially serious side effects. They are by prescription only, and for good reason. If you should, God forbid, get into a situation where you need to take anti-inflammatory steroids without medical supervision, you would definitely need to have some basic knowledge about them.

That being said, to take anti-inflammatory steroids for a couple of weeks in the face of an impending cytokine storm is quite reasonable. Many of the more serious side effects of anti-inflammatory steroids only occur over the longer term – months to years.

Understanding a Little More About Anti-Inflammatory Steroids

When talking about medicines we always talk about cautions, contraindications and side effects. Cautions are things about which you would be careful when using the medicine. Contraindications are when you would definitely not use the medicine. Side effects are things that you don't intend to happen from the medicine, but might happen anyway.

The cautions, contraindications and side effects of anti-inflammatory steroids are bewildering until their basic effects are understood. These steroids signal the body that there is an external, physical threat. The body prepares accordingly:

- Less energy goes to the immune system. The immune system is concerned with internal defense and clean-up. In an emergency, the body feels that this can wait.
  - For this reason, if there is already infection in the body (viruses, parasites, fungi) it may get worse. It's as if all the police rush to defend the borders, and the criminals

already within the borders are free to steal and loot.

- For this reason, they also recommend caution if the person may have a silent infection such as tuberculosis or parasites. They even caution use in people who have spent time in the tropics, where it's easy to contract parasites.
- For this reason they also recommend that you do not take live, attenuated vaccines while on anti-inflammatory steroids. (An attenuated vaccine is a vaccine where the germ or virus is alive but has been weakened.)
- And what's the point of taking any vaccine if your immune system is not going to respond? The function of anti-inflammatory steroids is to blunt the immune response.

- The blood pressure goes up: We need a full head of steam to deal with a physical emergency.
- The body holds in fluids: In an emergency you

may end up bleeding. Those fluids could be needed. Also, holding onto fluids helps to raise the blood pressure.

- The body holds onto sodium (salt) and dumps potassium. This is part of holding in fluids, but it can result in high sodium and low potassium in the blood, which make it hard for the body (especially the heart) to function properly.
- The blood sugar goes up: If we are going to run about and struggle physically for survival, we are going to need that sugar in the blood. If one already has diabetes, though, the diabetes could worsen.
- The blood flows away from the gut and to the animal brain, the muscles and the lungs. Basically the body says, "We can digest things later, after we survive this threat."
- This is part of the reason why the side effects of anti-inflammatory steroid use include ulcers and intestinal inflammation (colitis). If one already has either of these conditions, marked caution is indicated.
- Feeling crazy: It's easy to understand that the

ordinary, everyday state of mind in which we live is really quite different from the state of mind in which one would physically fight for one's life. Under threat, the spirit can become very agitated, which from the point of view of Western medicine becomes the possibilities of "euphoria, insomnia, mood swings, personality changes, severe depression, and frank psychotic manifestations"

- Increased pressure inside the eye (glaucoma).

Drug Interactions with Anti-Inflammatory Steroids

Drugs.com (http://drugs.com/) lists 498 possible drug interactions with methylprednisolone. They have a search function to see if your specific medication interacts. (https://www.drugs.com/drug-interactions/methylprednisolone.html)

While the specifics may be bewildering, they usually make sense once we understand the basic thrust of how anti-inflammatory steroids act. For example, if you are on high blood pressure medicine, the dosage may not be high enough if the anti-inflammatory steroids induce your body to retain water and drive the blood pressure up.

Also, just because there may be a drug-drug interaction, that does not necessarily mean one can't take the medicine. You might just need to adjust the dose, or watch that particular parameter. I would certainly accept, for example, a jump in blood pressure for a week while taking methylprednisolone over dying from the cytokine storm. And, if the vital signs are being followed, one would know to increase the blood pressure medicine as the blood pressure went up.

There is one other factor: medications are cleared from the body mostly by the liver and kidneys. Certain medications influence how quickly or slowly that occurs, which can mean that the doses of other medications have to be adjusted.

APPENDIX 6

Home Oxygen for Severe COVID-19

When the cytokine storm attacks the lungs, the lungs have trouble getting the oxygen out of the air. Without the oxygen, the body can't recover and heal. Oxygen is the basic energy currency on which our bodies run.

If you do not have oxygen on hand, you will certainly not be able to get it in a timely manner. At that point you are forced into going to the Emergency Room whether or not you would otherwise do so. Therefore if you do feel you may have trouble accessing medical care, or if you are severely opposed to going to the hospital, it would be good to have home oxygen on hand.

Recently, the FDA issued a specific warning against trying to use home oxygen for COVID-19, saying that it should only be used in the hospital. And it is true that too much oxygen can have its own bad effects on the lungs. But in moderate doses for a week or two, oxygen will do no harm. If I had worsening COVID-19 and couldn't get to a hospital, I wouldn't hesitate to use home oxygen until I could get help.

Concentrated oxygen is a powerful medicine. As with all medicines, the difference between healing and hurting is in the dose. With too much oxygen, lungs can become inflamed and scarred. The nervous system can become overstimulated, even to the point of seizures. But that is only when extremely high levels of oxygen are used.

The normal level of oxygen in the air at sea level is about 21% (the rest is mostly Nitrogen). The risk of inhaling a richer percentage of oxygen increases with the concentration of oxygen (up to 100%) and the time exposed.

Severe COVID-19 is a very temporary situation (whichever way it turns out). Home oxygen for a limited period of time is very unlikely to damage your lungs or nervous system. Ideally, you would have contact with a medical provider who could guide you in its use.

If you do have to use home oxygen and can't get medical guidance, my guideline would be to only take enough oxygen to bring your oxygen saturation up to 95%.

I recently attempted to get tanks of oxygen for a client to have at home just in case. I found it was not at all simple or easy. The medical system is set up to get you home oxygen on discharge from the hospital. The medical system is definitely not set up to get you home oxygen so that you don't have to go to the hospital in the first place.

However, there is an alternative to tanks for home oxygen. This is in the form of Home Oxygen Concentrators. They are machines that plug into house current. They contrate the oxygen that is already in the air.

As with pulse oximeters, there are Home Oxygen Concentrators that are medically approved and ones that are not medically approved. My impression is that the ones that are not medically approved are hastily-made, poorly constructed junk. Are they better than no oxygen concentrator at all? I don't know. (This is in contrast to my recommendations on non-FDA approved pulse oximeters: The non-FDA approved pulse oximeters do appear to be workable. The FDA-approved pulse oximeters are entirely unaffordable for most of us.)

A medically-approved oxygen concentrator would be much more reliable than one that is not approved. They are, of course, more expensive, and they require a doctor's prescription. You would need to find a doctor sympathetic to the needs of the current world situation. (And just forget about getting insurance to pay for it unless you already have a serious lung condition, documented by lung function tests).

APPENDIX 7

Blood Thinners (Anti-coagulants) to Prevent Clotting in Severe COVID-19

The cytokine storm is a form of extreme inflammation. With inflammation, the blood clots more easily. When the blood clots too much, blood flow is blocked and tissues don't receive the life-giving oxygen and nutrients they need. Therefore, when COVID-19 starts morphing into the cytokine storm, taking something to lessen how easily the blood clots is important.

In the hospital, they would give something like intravenous heparin, but that is not possible at home. (If the dose of Heparin is not just right, then the blood may become too thin and the person can start bleeding.)

The most common anti-coagulants that one can get over-the-counter are NSAIDs (Non-Seroidal Anti-Inflammatory Drugs) like Aspirin, Ibuprofen, Naproxen and so on.

For home use, Aspirin is the most commonly used anti-coagulant. The FLCCC recommends Aspirin 325 mg a day for early, out-patient COVID-19. Others recommend against this. If the experts can't agree, what is a humble General Practitioner to do?

When COVID-19 becomes severe and one adds anti-inflammatory steroids, there are cautions about possible interactions. Combining anti-inflammatory steroids with NSAIDs may increase the risk of stomach and intestinal ulcers and bleeding. So there is debate on whether or not one should take these two medicines together in the setting of severe COVID-19.

If the cytokine storm is life-threatening, one is going to need pharmaceutical blood thinners under supervision in a hospital environment. This is one reason why severe COVID-19 needs to be handled in the hospital.

But until one has arrived at the hospital, I wouldn't hesitate to intensify the measures to reduce clotting described on page 34 in Chapter 6.

Again, though, please remember that the difference between a medicine and a poison is only in the dose. Use judgement and common sense, and don't overdo it.

APPENDIX 8

Shopping List for COVID-19 Preparedness

You want to lay in your supplies before you or a loved one falls ill from COVID-19. It would be heartbreaking to have to rush about in a panic once someone is already ill, finding out that the supply chain and the medical system is not as forthcoming as you might imagine.

Get from the store or online:

Equipment

- ☐ Pulse oximeter (this is the key piece of equipment)
- ☐ Blood pressure cuff
- ☐ Thermometer

Medicines

- ☐ Zinc
- ☐ Quercetin
- ☐ Vitamin D
- ☐ Melatonin

Get from a Physician

- ☐ Ivermectin

(Please see **APPENDIX 2: Obtaining Ivermectin** for possible places).

I recommend you lay in at a minimum 5 of the 12 mg tablets for each adult in the house.

Optional Stuff

- ☐ Anti-inflammatory steroids
- ☐ Home oxygen concentrator—need a physician prescription.

(Please see **APPENDIX 6: Home Oxygen for Severe COVID-19**)

APPENDIX 9

The HCQ (Hydroxychloroquine) Approach

Early in the epidemic there was fierce debate about re-purposing a medicine called Hydroxychloroquine, which I will refer to as "HCQ. "Re-purposing" is the idea that we could take a medicine we already know is safe and FDA-approved and use it for some other illness than the one for which it was originally approved. HCQ was a great possibility because it is inexpensive and out of patent. It is normally used for rheumatoid arthritis, lupus and malaria.

HCQ's advocates were Harvey Risch, MD and Vladimir Zelenko, MD. They both insisted on one point which was lost in the subsequent frenzy of political smearing. That one point is that *HCQ is proven useful for COVID-19 in one specific situation: a high-risk person early in the illness*.

Some other sources advocate it for other situations, but the specific usage above is the one about which I am convinced.

The details of the HCQ approach vary by time and author, but here are the essentials for the early outpatient treatment of COVID-19 as outlined by Vladimir Zelenko, MD:

1. Anyone with shortness of breath is treated immediately.

2. Anyone with mild symptoms who is high-risk is treated immediately.

3. The regimen is:

- **HCQ (Hydroxychloroquine)** 200 mg by mouth twice daily for five days.
- (If HCQ is unavailable, **Quercetin** serves a similar function)
- **Azithromycin** 500 mg once a day for five days (Azithromycin is an antibiotic)
- **Zinc Sulfate** 50 mg (of elemental Zinc) a day for 5 days.

Dr. Zelenko has had wonderful results with this protocol.

https://www.sciencedirect.com/science/article/pii/S0924857920304258

References

The references in this section pertain to COVID-19. Many, but not all, of them pertain to Ivermectin. Other studies, as for example on the use of Vitamin D to prevent COVID-19, are included.

The Frontline COVID-19 Critical Care Alliance has produced a position paper titled:

"*Review of the Emerging Evidence Demonstrating the Efficacy of Ivermectin in the Prophylaxis and Treatment of COVID-19.*"

It was the references in this paper that convinced me, and I reproduce them below in their entirety.

If you have been convinced that Ivermectin has an important role in ending the COVID-19 epidemic, I encourage you to download this, print out a copy and give it to your doctor.

https://covid19criticalcare.com/wp-content/uploads/2020/11/FLCCC-Ivermectin-in-the-prophylaxis-and-treatment-of-COVID-19.pdf

If you would like a more complete list of 464 references on COVID-19, you can go to:

https://covid19criticalcare.com/wp-content/uploads/2020/12/FLCCC-Protocols-—-A-Guide-to-the-Management-of-COVID-19.pdf

Since our knowledge about the treatment of COVID-19 is in constant evolution, there is also a website that keeps an up-to-date list of studies on drugs used to treat COVID-19, including Ivermectin, Vitamin D, Hydroxychloroquine and more. You can find that here:

https://c19early.com/

Them that have eyes, let them read.

References from "*Review of the Emerging Evidence Demonstrating the Efficacy of Ivermectin in the Prophylaxis and Treatment of COVID-19.*"

https://covid19criticalcare.com/wp-content/uploads/2020/11/FLCCC-Ivermectin-in-the-prophylaxis-and-treatment-of-COVID-19.pdf)

1. Agarwal, A., Mukherjee, A., Kumar, G., Chatterjee, P., Bhatnagar, T., Malhotra, P., and Collaborators, P.T. (2020). Convalescent plasma in the management of moderate COVID-19 in adults in India: open label phase II multicentre randomised controlled trial (PLACID Trial). *BMJ* 371, m3939.
2. Aguirre-Chang, G. (2020). Post-Acute or prolonged COVID-19: treatment with Ivermectin for patients with persistent, or post-acute symptoms *ResearchGate*.
3. Ahmed, S., Karim, M.M., Ross, A.G., Hossain, M.S., Clemens, J.D., Sumiya, M.K., Phru, C.S., Rahman, M., Zaman, K., and Somani, J. (2020). A five day course of Ivermectin for the treatment of COVID-19 may reduce the duration of illness. *International Journal of Infectious Diseases*.

4. Alam, M., R, M., Pf, G., Md, M.Z., S, S., and Ma, C. (2020). Ivermectin as Pre-exposure Prophylaxis for COVID-19 among Healthcare Providers in a Selected Tertiary Hospital in Dhaka An Observational Study. *European Journal of Medical and Health Sciences*.
5. Anglemyer, A., Horvath, H.T., and Bero, L. (2014). Healthcare outcomes assessed with observational study designs compared with those assessed in randomized trials. *Cochrane Database Syst Rev*, MR000034.
6. Arevalo, A.P., Pagotto, R., Porfido, J., Daghero, H., Segovia, M., Yamasaki, K., Varela, B., Hill, M., Verdes, J.M., and Vega, MD (2020). Ivermectin reduces coronavirus infection in vivo: a mouse experimental model. *bioRxiv*.
7. Atkinson, S.C., Audsley, MD, Lieu, K.G., Marsh, G.A., Thomas, D.R., Heaton, S.M., Paxman, J.J., Wagstaff, K.M., Buckle, A.M., Moseley, G.W., Jans, D.A., and Borg, N.A. (2018). Recognition by host nuclear transport proteins drives disorder-to-order transition in Hendra virus V. *Scientific Reports* 8, 358.

8. Babalola, O.E., Bode, C.O., Ajayi, A.A., Alakaloko, F.M., Akase, I.E., Otrofanowei, E., Salu, O.B., Adeyemo, W.L., Ademuyiwa, A.O., and Omilabu, S.A. Ivermectin shows clinical benefits in mild to moderate COVID-19 disease: A randomised controlled double blind dose response study in Lagos. *medRxiv*, 2021.2001. 2005.21249131.
9. Behera, P., Patro, B.K., Singh, A.K., Chandanshive, P.D., Ravikumar, S., Pradhan, S.K., Pentapati, S.S.K., Batmanabane, G., Padhy, B.M., and Bal, S. (2020). Role of Ivermectin in the prevention of COVID-19 infection among healthcare workers in India: A matched case-control study. *medRxiv*.
10. Bernigaud, C., Guillemot, D., Ahmed-Belkacem, A., Grimaldi-Bensouda, L., Lespine, A., Berry, F., Softic, L., Chenost, C., Do-Pham, G., and Giraudeau, B. (Year). "Bénéfice de l'Ivermectine: de la gale à la COVID-19, un exemple de sérendipité", in: *Annales de Dermatologie et de Vénéréologie*: Elsevier), A194.

11. Bray, M., Rayner, C., Noël, F., Jans, D., and Wagstaff, K. (2020). Ivermectin and COVID-19: a report in Antiviral Research, widespread interest, an FDA warning, two letters to the editor and the authors' responses. *Antiviral Research.*
12. Budhiraja, S., Soni, A., Jha, V., Indrayan, A., Dewan, A., Singh, O., Singh, Y., Chugh, I., Arora, V., and Pandey, R. (2020). Clinical Profile of First 1000 COVID-19 Cases Admitted at Tertiary Care Hospitals and the Correlates of their Mortality: An Indian Experience. *medRxiv.*
13. Cadegiani, F.A., Goren, A., Wambier, C.G., and Mccoy, J. (2020). Early COVID-19 Therapy with Azithromycin Plus Nitazoxanide, Ivermectin or Hydroxychloroquine in Outpatient Settings Significantly Reduced Symptoms Compared to Known Outcomes in Untreated Patients. *medRxiv.*
14. Callard, F., and Perego, E. (2020). How and why patients made Long COVID-19. *Social Science & Medicine*, 113426.

15. Caly, L., Druce, J.D., Catton, M.G., Jans, D.A., and Wagstaff, K.M. (2020a). The FDA-approved drug Ivermectin inhibits the replication of SARS-CoV-2 in vitro. *Antiviral Res* 178, 104787
16. Caly, L., Druce, J.D., Catton, M.G., Jans, D.A., and Wagstaff, K.M. (2020b). The FDA-approved drug Ivermectin inhibits the replication of SARS-CoV-2 in vitro. *Antiviral Research* 178, 104787.
17. Carvallo, H.E., Hirsch, R.R., and Farinella, M.E. (2020a). Safety and Efficacy of the combined use of Ivermectin, dexamethasone, enoxaparin and aspirin against COVID-19. *medRxiv*.
18. Carvallo, H.E., Roberto, H., Psaltis, A., and Veronica, C. (2020b). Study of the Efficacy and Safety of Topical Ivermectin+ Iota-Carrageenan in the Prophylaxis against COVID-19 in Health Personnel.

19. Chaccour, C., Casellas, A., Blanco-Di Matteo, A., Pineda, I., Fernandez-Montero, A., Castillo, P.R., Richardson, M.-A., Mateos, M.R., Jordan-Iborra, C., and Brew, J. (2020). The effect of early treatment with Ivermectin on viral load, symptoms and humoral response in patients with mild COVID-19: a pilot, double-blind, placebo-controlled, randomized clinical trial.
20. Chachar, A.Z.K., Khan, K.A., Asif, M., Tanveer, K., Khaqan, A., and Basri, R. (2020). Effectiveness of Ivermectin in SARS-CoV-2/ COVID-19 Patients. *International Journal of Sciences* 9, 31-35.
21. Chala (2020). Prophylaxis COVID-19 in Healthcare Agents by Intensive Treatment With Ivermectin and Iota-carrageenan (Ivercar-Tuc). *ClinicalTrials.gov* NCT04701710.
22. Chamie, J. (2020). *Real-World Evidence: The Case of Peru. Causality between Ivermectin and COVID-19 Infection Fatality Rate.*

23. Chandler, R.E. (2018). Serious neurological adverse events after Ivermectin—do they occur beyond the indication of onchocerciasis? *The American journal of tropical medicine and hygiene* 98, 382-388.
24. Chowdhury, A.T.M.M., Shahbaz, M., Karim, M.R., Islam, J., Guo, D., and He, S. (2020). A Randomized Trial of Ivermectin-Doxycycline and Hydroxychloroquine-Azithromycin therapy on COVID-1919 patients.
25. Ci, X., Li, H., Yu, Q., Zhang, X., Yu, L., Chen, N., Song, Y., and Deng, X. (2009). Avermectin exerts anti-inflammatory effect by downregulating the nuclear transcription factor kappa-B and mitogen-activated protein kinase activation pathway. *Fundam Clin Pharmacol* 23, 449-455.
26. Consortium, W.S.T. (2020). Repurposed antiviral drugs for COVID-19—interim WHO SOLIDARITY trial results. medRxiv. *Preprint posted online* 15.

27. Crump, A., and Omura, S. (2011). Ivermectin,'wonder drug' from Japan: the human use perspective. *Proceedings of the Japan Academy, Series B* 87, 13-28.
28. Dahabreh, I.J., Sheldrick, R.C., Paulus, J.K., Chung, M., Varvarigou, V., Jafri, H., Rassen, J.A., Trikalinos, T.A., and Kitsios, G.D. (2012). Do observational studies using propensity score methods agree with randomized trials? A systematic comparison of studies on acute coronary syndromes. *European Heart Journal* 33, 1893-1901.
29. Dasgupta J, S.U., Bakshi a, Dasgupta a, Manna K, Saha, C De, Rk, Mukhopadhyay S, Bhattacharyya Np (2020). Nsp7 and Spike Glycoprotein of SARS-CoV-2 Are Envisaged as Potential Targets of Vitamin D and Ivermectin. *Preprints*.
30. Dayer, M.R. (2020). Coronavirus (2019-nCoV) Deactivation via Spike Glycoprotein Shielding by Old Drugs, Bioinformatic Study.

31. De Melo, G.D., Lazarini, F., Larrous, F., Feige, L., Kergoat, L., Marchio, A., Pineau, P., Lecuit, M., Lledo, P.-M., Changeux, J.-P., and Bourhy, H. (2020). Anti-COVID-19 efficacy of Ivermectin in the golden hamster. *bioRxiv*, 2020.2011.2021.392639.
32. Elgazzar, A., Hany, B., Youssef, S.A., Hafez, M., and Moussa, H. (2020). Efficacy and Safety of Ivermectin for Treatment and prophylaxis of COVID-19 Pandemic.
33. Entrenas Castillo, M., Entrenas Costa, L.M., Vaquero Barrios, J.M., Alcala Diaz, J.F., Lopez Miranda, J., Bouillon, R., and Quesada Gomez, J.M. (2020). "Effect of calcifediol treatment and best available therapy versus best available therapy on intensive care unit admission and mortality among patients hospitalized for COVID-19: A pilot randomized clinical study". *J Steroid Biochem Mol Biol* 203, 105751.

34. Espitia-Hernandez, G., Munguia, L., Diaz-Chiguer, D., Lopez-Elizalde, R., and Jimenez-Ponce, F. (2020). Effects of Ivermectin-azithromycin-cholecalciferol combined therapy on COVID-19 infected patients: a proof of concept study.
35. Gardon, J., Gardon-Wendel, N., Demanga, N., Kamgno, J., Chippaux, J.-P., and Boussinesq, M. (1997). Serious reactions after mass treatment of onchocerciasis with Ivermectin in an area endemic for Loa loa infection. *The Lancet* 350, 18-22.
36. Gorial, F.I., Mashhadani, S., Sayaly, H.M., Dakhil, B.D., Almashhadani, M.M., Aljabory, A.M., Abbas, Hassan M, Ghanim, M., and Rasheed, J.I. (2020). Effectiveness of Ivermectin as add-on Therapy in COVID-19 Management (Pilot Trial). *medRxiv*.

37. Götz, V., Magar, L., Dornfeld, D., Giese, S., Pohlmann, A., Höper, D., Kong, B.-W., Jans, D.A., Beer, M., Haller, O., and Schwemmle, M. (2016). Influenza A viruses escape from MxA restriction at the expense of efficient nuclear vRNP import. *Scientific Reports* 6, 23138.
38. Guzzo, C., Furtek, C., Porras, A., Chen, C., Tipping, R., Clineschmidt, C., Sciberras, D., Hsieh, J., and Lasseter, K. (2002). Safety, Tolerability, and Pharmacokinetics of Escalating High Doses of Ivermectin in Healthy Adult Subjects. *Journal of clinical pharmacology* 42, 1122-1133.
39. Hashim, H.A., Maulood, M.F., Rasheed, A.M., Fatak, D.F., Kabah, K.K., and Abdulamir, A.S. (2020). Controlled randomized clinical trial on using Ivermectin with Doxycycline for treating COVID-19 patients in Baghdad, Iraq. *medRxiv*.
40. Hellwig, MD, and Maia, A. (2020). A COVID-19 Prophylaxis? Lower incidence associated with prophylactic administration of Ivermectin. *Int J Antimicrob Agents*, 106248.

41. Hermine, O., Mariette, X., Tharaux, P.L., Resche-Rigon, M., Porcher, R., Ravaud, P., and Group, C.-C. (2020). Effect of Tocilizumab vs Usual Care in Adults Hospitalized With COVID-19 and Moderate or Severe Pneumonia: A Randomized Clinical Trial. *JAMA Intern Med.*
42. Horby, P., Lim, W.S., Emberson, J.R., Mafham, M., Bell, J.L., Linsell, L., Staplin, N., Brightling, C., Ustianowski, A., and Elmahi, E. (2020). Dexamethasone in hospitalized patients with COVID-19-preliminary report. *The New England journal of medicine*.
43. Hussien, M.A., and Abdelaziz, A.E. (2020). Molecular docking suggests repurposing of brincidofovir as a potential drug targeting SARS-CoV-2 ACE2 receptor and main protease. *Network Modeling Analysis in Health Informatics and Bioinformatics* 9, 1-18.
44. Jehi, L., Ji, X., Milinovich, A., Erzurum, S., Rubin, B.P., Gordon, S., Young, J.B., and Kattan, M.W. (2020). Individualizing Risk Prediction for Positive Coronavirus Disease 2019 Testing: Results From 11,672 Patients. *Chest* 158, 1364-1375.

45. Kalfas, S., Visvanathan, K., Chan, K., and Drago, J. (2020). THE THERAPEUTIC POTENTIAL OF IVERMECTIN FOR COVID-19: A REVIEW OF MECHANISMS AND EVIDENCE. *medRxiv*.
46. Khan, M.S.I., Khan, M.S.I., Debnath, C.R., Nath, P.N., Mahtab, M.A., Nabeka, H., Matsuda, S., and Akbar, S.M.F. (2020). Ivermectin Treatment May Improve the Prognosis of Patients With COVID-19. *Archivos de Bronconeumología*.
47. King, C.R., Tessier, T.M., Dodge, M.J., Weinberg, J.B., and Mymryk, J.S. (2020). Inhibition of Human Adenovirus Replication by the Importin α/β1 Nuclear Import Inhibitor Ivermectin. *Journal of Virology* 94.
48. Kircik, L.H., Del Rosso, J.Q., Layton, A.M., and Schauber, J. (2016). Over 25 Years of Clinical Experience With Ivermectin: An Overview of Safety for an Increasing Number of Indications. Journal of drugs in dermatology : JDD 15, 325-332.

49. Kitsios, G.D., Dahabreh, I.J., Callahan, S., Paulus, J.K., Campagna, A.C., and Dargin, J.M. (2015). Can We Trust Observational Studies Using Propensity Scores in the Critical Care Literature? A Systematic Comparison With Randomized Clinical Trials. *Crit Care Med* 43, 1870-1879.
50. Kory, P., Meduri, G.U., Iglesias, J., Varon, J., and Marik, P.E. (2020). Clinical and Scientific Rationale for the "MATH+" Hospital Treatment Protocol for COVID-19. *Journal of Intensive Care Medicine*.
51. Lehrer, S., and Rheinstein, P.H. (2020). Ivermectin Docks to the SARS-CoV-2 Spike Receptor-binding Domain Attached to ACE2. *In Vivo* 34, 3023-3026.
52. Li, Y., Chen, M., Cao, H., Zhu, Y., Zheng, J., and Zhou, H. (2013). Extraordinary GU-rich single-strand RNA identified from SARS coronavirus contributes an excessive innate immune response. *Microbes Infect* 15, 88-95.

53. Lonjon, G., Boutron, I., Trinquart, L., Ahmad, N., Aim, F., Nizard, R., and Ravaud, P. (2014). Comparison of treatment effect estimates from prospective nonrandomized studies with propensity score analysis and randomized controlled trials of surgical procedures. *Ann Surg 259, 18-25.*
54. Lv, C., Liu, W., Wang, B., Dang, R., Qiu, L., Ren, J., Yan, C., Yang, Z., and Wang, X. (2018). Ivermectin inhibits DNA polymerase UL42 of pseudorabies virus entrance into the nucleus and proliferation of the virus in vitro and vivo. *Antiviral Research* 159, 55-62.
55. Mahmud, R. (2020). A Randomized, Double-Blind Placebo Controlled Clinical Trial of Ivermectin plus Doxycycline for the Treatment of Confirmed COVID-19 Infection.
56. Marik, P.E., Kory, P., Varon, J., Iglesias, J., and Meduri, G.U. (2020). MATH+ protocol for the treatment of SARS-CoV-2 infection: the scientific rationale. *Expert Review of Anti-infective Therapy*, 1-7.

57. Mastrangelo, E., Pezzullo, M., De Burghgraeve, T., Kaptein, S., Pastorino, B., Dallmeier, K., De Lamballerie, X., Neyts, J., Hanson, A.M., Frick, D.N., Bolognesi, M., and Milani, M. (2012). Ivermectin is a potent inhibitor of flavivirus replication specifically targeting NS3 helicase activity: new prospects for an old drug. *Journal of Antimicrobial Chemotherapy* 67, 1884-1894.
58. Maurya, D.K. (2020). A combination of Ivermectin and doxycycline possibly blocks the viral entry and modulate the innate immune response in COVID-19 patients.
59. Morgenstern, J., Redondo, J.N., De Leon, A., Canela, J.M., Torres, N., Tavares, J., Minaya, M., Lopez, O., Placido, A.M., and Castillo, A. (2020). The use of compassionate Ivermectin in the management of symptomatic outpatients and hospitalized patients with clinical diagnosis of COVID-19 at the Medical Center Bournigal and the Medical Center Punta Cana, Rescue Group, Dominican Republic, from may 1 to august 10, 2020. *medRxiv*.

60. Nadkarni, G.N., Lala, A., Bagiella, E., Chang, H.L., Moreno, P.R., Pujadas, E., Arvind, V., Bose, S., Charney, A.W., Chen, MD, Cordon-Cardo, C., Dunn, A.S., Farkouh, M.E., Glicksberg, B.S., Kia, A., Kohli-Seth, R., Levin, M.A., Timsina, P., Zhao, S., Fayad, Z.A., and Fuster, V. (2020). Anticoagulation, Bleeding, Mortality, and Pathology in Hospitalized Patients With COVID-19. *J Am Coll Cardiol* 76, 1815-1826.
61. Nallusamy, S., Mannu, J., Ravikumar, C., Angamuthu, K., Nathan, B., Nachimuthu, K., Ramasamy, G., Muthurajan, R., Subbarayalu, M., and Neelakandan, K. (2020). Shortlisting Phytochemicals Exhibiting Inhibitory Activity against Major Proteins of SARS-CoV-2 through Virtual Screening.
62. Niaee, M.S., Gheibi, N., Namdar, P., Allami, A., Zolghadr, L., Javadi, A., Karampour, A., Varnaseri, M., Bizhani, B., and Cheraghi, F. (2020). Ivermectin as an adjunct treatment for hospitalized adult COVID-19 patients: A randomized multi-center clinical trial.

63. Perera, R.A., Tso, E., Tsang, O.T., Tsang, D.N., Fung, K., Leung, Y.W., Chin, A.W., Chu, D.K., Cheung, S.M., and Poon, L.L. (2020). SARS-CoV-2 virus culture from the upper respiratory tract: Correlation with viral load, subgenomic viral RNA and duration of illness. *MedRXiv*.
64. Podder, C.S., Chowdhury, N., Sina, M.I., and Haque, W. (2020). Outcome of Ivermectin treated mild to moderate COVID-19 cases: a single-centre, open-label, randomised controlled study. *IMC J. Med. Sci* 14.
65. Polak, S.B., Van Gool, I.C., Cohen, D., Von Der Thusen, J.H., and Van Paassen, J. (2020). A systematic review of pathological findings in COVID-19: a pathophysiological timeline and possible mechanisms of disease progression. *Mod Pathol* 33, 2128-2138.
66. Portmann-Baracco, A., Bryce-Alberti, M., and Accinelli, R.A. (2020). Antiviral and Anti-Inflammatory Properties of Ivermectin and Its Potential Use in COVID-19. *Arch Bronconeumol*.

67. Rajter, J.C., Sherman, M.S., Fatteh, N., Vogel, F., Sacks, J., and Rajter, J.J. (2020). Use of Ivermectin is Associated with Lower Mortality in Hospitalized Patients with COVID-19 (ICON study). *Chest*.
68. Ravikirti, Roy, R., Pattadar, C., Raj, R., Agarwal, N., Biswas, B., Majhi, P.K., Rai, D.K., Shyama, Kumar, A., and Sarfaraz, A. (2021). Ivermectin as a potential treatment for mild to moderate COVID-19 – A double blind randomized placebo-controlled trial. *medRxiv*, 2021.2001.2005.21249310.
69. Robin, R.C., Alam, R.F., Saber, S., Bhiuyan, E., Murshed, R., and Alam, M.T. (2020). A Case Series of 100 COVID-19 Positive Patients Treated with Combination of Ivermectin and Doxycycline. *Journal of Bangladesh College of Physicians and Surgeons*, 10-15.
70. Rodriguez-Nava, G., Trelles-Garcia, D.P., Yanez-Bello, M.A., Chung, C.W., Trelles-Garcia, V.P., and Friedman, H.J. (2020). Atorvastatin associated with decreased hazard for death in COVID-19 patients admitted to an ICU: a retrospective cohort study. *Crit Care* 24, 429.

71. Rubin, R. (2020). As Their Numbers Grow, COVID-19 “Long Haulers” Stump Experts. *JAMA* 324, 1381-1383.
72. Salvarani, C., Dolci, G., Massari, M., Merlo, D.F., Cavuto, S., Savoldi, L., Bruzzi, P., Boni, F., Braglia, L., Turra, C., Ballerini, P.F., Sciascia, R., Zammarchi, L., Para, O., Scotton, P.G., Inojosa, W.O., Ravagnani, V., Salerno, N.D., Sainaghi, P.P., Brignone, A., Codeluppi, M., Teopompi, E., Milesi, M., Bertomoro, P., Claudio, N., Salio, M., Falcone, M., Cenderello, G., Donghi, L., Del Bono, V., Colombelli, P.L., Angheben, A., Passaro, A., Secondo, G., Pascale, R., Piazza, I., Facciolongo, N., Costantini, M., and Group, R.-T.-C.-S. (2020). Effect of Tocilizumab vs Standard Care on Clinical Worsening in Patients Hospitalized With COVID-19 Pneumonia: A Randomized Clinical Trial. *JAMA Intern Med*
73. Scheim, D. (2020). “From Cold to Killer: How SARS-CoV-2 Evolved without Hemagglutinin Esterase to Agglutinate, Then Clot Blood Cells in Pulmonary and Systemic Microvasculature”. SSRN).

74. Schmith, V.D., Zhou, J., and Lohmer, L.R. (2020). The Approved Dose of Ivermectin Alone is not the Ideal Dose for the Treatment of COVID-19. *Clinical Pharmacology & Therapeutics*.
75. Sen Gupta, P.S., Biswal, S., Panda, S.K., Ray, A.K., and Rana, M.K. (2020). Binding mechanism and structural insights into the identified protein target of COVID-19 and importin-alpha with in-vitro effective drug Ivermectin. *J Biomol Struct Dyn*, 1-10.
76. Shouman, W. (2020). Use of Ivermectin as a Prophylactic Option in Asymptomatic Family Close Contact for Patient with COVID-19. *Clincal Trials.gov*.
77. Siegelman, J.N. (2020). Reflections of a COVID-19 Long Hauler. *JAMA*.

78. Soto-Becerra, P., Culquichicón, C., Hurtado-Roca, Y., and Araujo-Castillo, R.V. (2020). Real-world effectiveness of hydroxychloroquine, azithromycin, and Ivermectin among hospitalized COVID-19 patients: results of a target trial emulation using observational data from a nationwide healthcare system in Peru. *Azithromycin, and Ivermectin Among Hospitalized COVID-19 Patients: Results of a Target Trial Emulation Using Observational Data from a Nationwide Healthcare System in Peru.*
79. Sparsa, A., Bonnetblanc, J., Peyrot, I., Loustaud-Ratti, V., Vidal, E., and Bedane, C. (Year). "Systemic adverse reactions with Ivermectin treatment of scabies", in: *Annales de Dermatologie et de Venereologie*), 784-787.
80. Spoorthi V, S.S. (2020). Utility of Ivermectin and Doxycycline combination for the treatment of SARS-CoV2. *International Archives of Integrated Medicine* 7, 177-182.

81. Suravajhala, R., Parashar, A., Malik, B., Nagaraj, A.V., Padmanaban, G., Kishor, P.K., Polavarapu, R., and Suravajhala, P. (2020). Comparative Docking Studies on Curcumin with COVID-19 Proteins.
82. Swargiary, A. (2020). Ivermectin as a promising RNA-dependent RNA polymerase inhibitor and a therapeutic drug against SARS-CoV2: Evidence from in silico studies.
83. Tambo, E., Khater, E.I., Chen, J.H., Bergquist, R., and Zhou, X.N. Nobel prize for the artemisinin and Ivermectin discoveries: a great boost towards elimination of the global infectious diseases of poverty.
84. Tay, M.Y.F., Fraser, J.E., Chan, W.K.K., Moreland, N.J., Rathore, A.P., Wang, C., Vasudevan, S.G., and Jans, D.A. (2013). Nuclear localization of dengue virus (DENV) 1–4 non-structural protein 5; protection against all 4 DENV serotypes by the inhibitor Ivermectin. *Antiviral Research* 99, 301-306.

85. Varghese, F.S., Kaukinen, P., Gläsker, S., Bespalov, M., Hanski, L., Wennerberg, K., Kümmerer, B.M., and Ahola, T. (2016). Discovery of berberine, abamectin and Ivermectin as antivirals against chikungunya and other alphaviruses. *Antiviral Research* 126, 117-124.
86. Veit, O., Beck, B., Steuerwald, M., and Hatz, C. (2006). First case of Ivermectin-induced severe hepatitis. *Transactions of the Royal Society of Tropical Medicine and Hygiene* 100, 795-797.
87. Wagstaff, Kylie m., Sivakumaran, H., Heaton, Steven m., Harrich, D., and Jans, David a. (2012). Ivermectin is a specific inhibitor of importin α/β-mediated nuclear import able to inhibit replication of HIV-1 and dengue virus. *Biochemical Journal* 443, 851-856.
88. Yang, S.N.Y., Atkinson, S.C., Wang, C., Lee, A., Bogoyevitch, M.A., Borg, N.A., and Jans, D.A. (2020). The broad spectrum antiviral Ivermectin targets the host nuclear transport importin α/β1 heterodimer. *Antiviral Research* 177, 104760.

89. Young, B.E., Ong, S.W., Ng, L.F., Anderson, D.E., Chia, W.N., Chia, P.Y., Ang, L.W., Mak, T.-M., Kalimuddin, S., and Chai, L.Y.A. (2020). Viral dynamics and immune correlates of COVID-19 disease severity. *Clinical infectious diseases: an official publication of the Infectious Diseases Society of America.*
90. Zhang, J., Rao, X., Li, Y., Zhu, Y., Liu, F., Guo, G., Luo, G., Meng, Z., De Backer, D., and Xiang, H. (2020a). High-dose vitamin C infusion for the treatment of critically ill COVID-19.
91. Zhang, X., Song, Y., Ci, X., An, N., Ju, Y., Li, H., Wang, X., Han, C., Cui, J., and Deng, X. (2008). Ivermectin inhibits LPS-induced production of inflammatory cytokines and improves LPS-induced survival in mice. *Inflamm Res* 57, 524-529.
92. Zhang, X., Song, Y., Xiong, H., Ci, X., Li, H., Yu, L., Zhang, L., and Deng, X. (2009). Inhibitory effects of Ivermectin on nitric oxide and prostaglandin E2 production in LPS-stimulated RAW 264.7 macrophages. *Int Immunopharmacol* 9, 354-359.

93. Zhang, X.-J., Qin, J.-J., Cheng, X., Shen, L., Zhao, Y.-C., Yuan, Y., Lei, F., Chen, M.-M., Yang, H., and Bai, L. (2020b). In-hospital use of statins is associated with a reduced risk of mortality among individuals with COVID-19. *Cell metabolism* 32, 176-187. e174

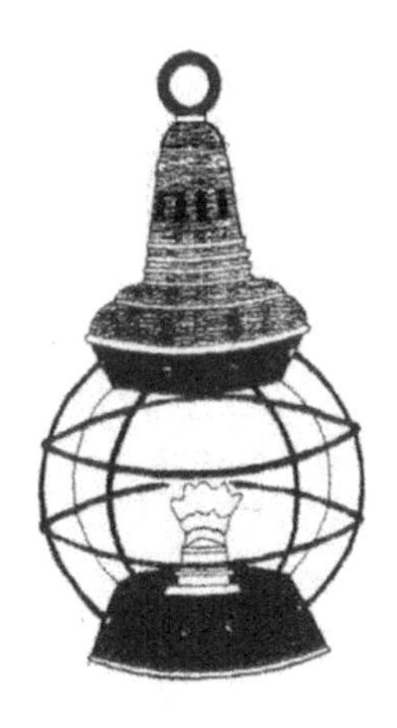

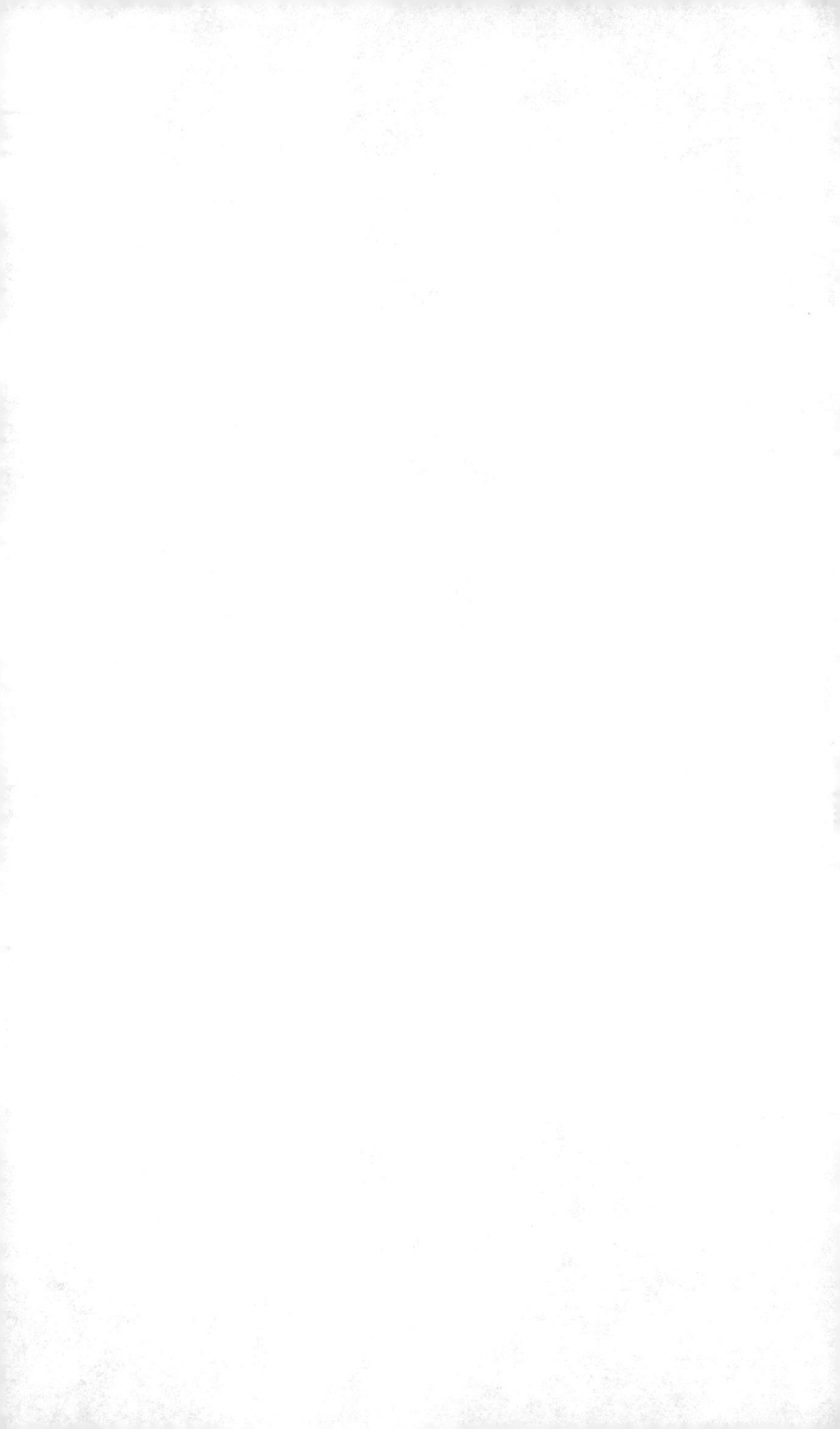

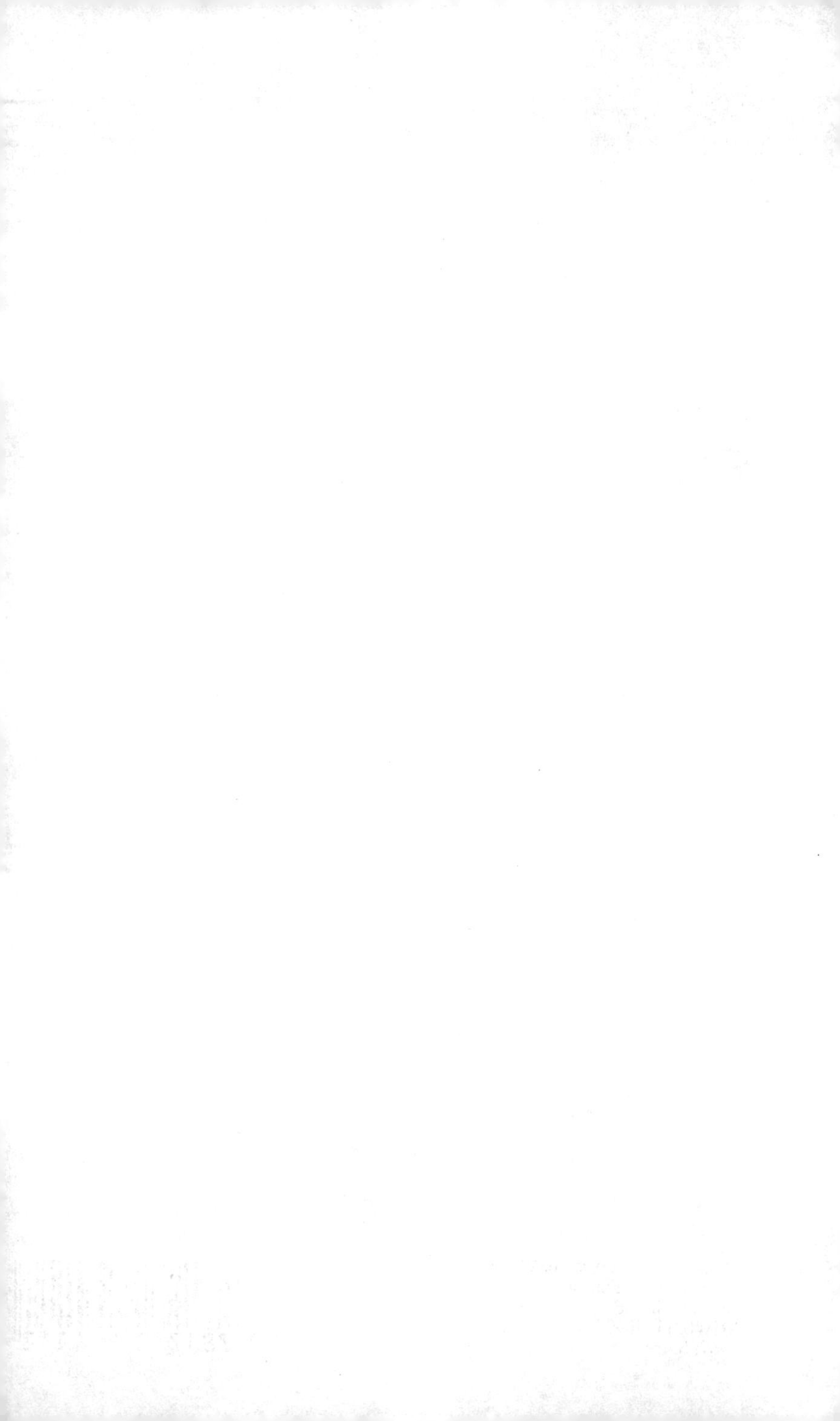

CPSIA information can be obtained
at www.ICGtesting.com
Printed in the USA
FSHW021107090721
82967FS

9 781732 104112